May the journey into your own personal discovery be a gentle wisdom into health & vitality. Life is meant to be fun. Remember you always have permission to heal in your own time & space. Once we get out of our own road, the universe conspires to help us in every way possible.

"Love This Life"

Ranee Zeller

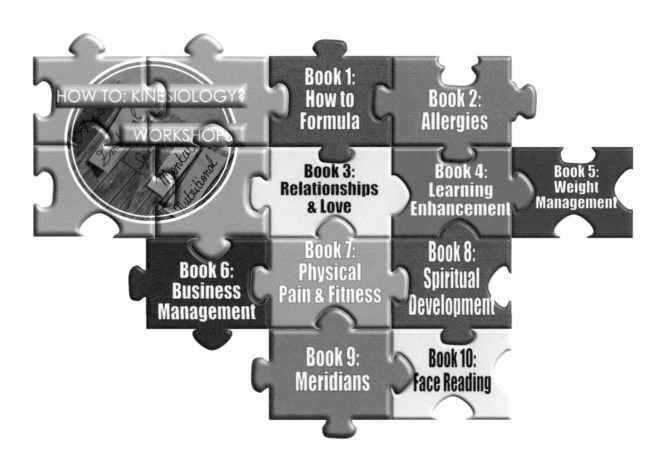

PERSONAL & PROFESSIONAL DEVELOPMENT ECO RETREATS

At Bayside Kinesiology we have the perfect environment for Organisational Team Building workshops. We offer a range of unique educational experiences allowing a whole paradigm shift to evolve within your personal or work/club teams. With over 20 years experience in communication, natural and remedial therapies we can offer you professional development and support in a caring environment.

After arriving at Brisbane domestic or international airport you will be transported to our tranquil Australian bushland setting.

We offer the whole package education, team challenges, relaxation, food, accommodation and airport pickups.

We can tailor individual packages just for your circumstances or you can either choose from our range of established packages or design your own.

For information or to contact us

Phone:	+61 7 32060421
Text:	+61 419 737 396
Web:	www.baysidekinesiology.com
Email:	ranee.zeller@baysidekinesiology.com
FB:	Bayside Kinesiology
Skype:	Ranee Zeller

INDEX

DISCLAIMER STATEMENT

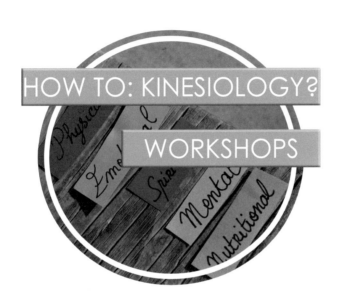

ABOUT THE AUTHOR

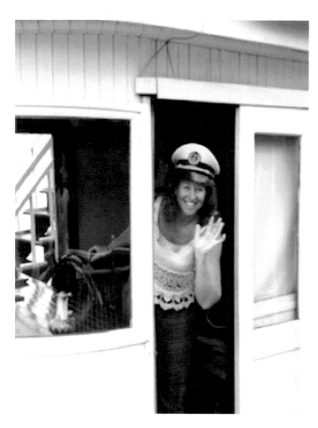

Born in Queensland, Australia, Ranee Zeller holds diplomas in Kinesiology, massage, sport & fitness, hotel management, certificates in childcare, and a Level 1 Yoga Instructor. Ranee's early background was in children's day care. During this time she developed in-depth insights into early childhood thought, learning and development, as well as family and group dynamics. She has been lecturing in and practicing Kinesiology since 1994 and now she is also a massage therapist, reflexologist, Kinergetics instructor and Jaw R. E. S. E. T. instructor. She has worked on everyone from Para-Olympians and sports athletes to scientists, artists, autistic children and business professionals.

Ranee has also been fortunate to help alleviate the suffering of those battling fibromyalgia, cancer and other illnesses.

Ranee and her family constantly strive to improve their permaculture property. Their live-in retreats include a real education on health, vitality and natural therapies education.

In 1996, Ranee began to create her "HOW TO Kinesiology" formula which is appropriate for

- Educational teachers/lecturers/students
- Medical students
- Natural therapists
- General public
- Yoga Instructors

Introduction Video on YouTube
https//www.youtube.com/watch?v=_0Pmzm_3pGU

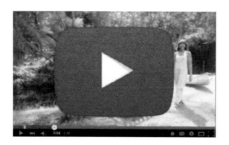

INTRODUCTION

When doing kinesiology testing you are testing the energy imbalance in relation to that one specific question that links to how it is in the present moment. Once it has been identified on the energy level you MUST be very specific about your questioning. The more detailed you can be the more accurate the answer. For example: how often, how long, how much, when and where are all extremely important to the accuracy of kinesiology testing.

THE ORIGIN OF KINESIOLOGY

Kinesiology began in the 20th century by orthopaedic surgeon Robert W. Lovett who first pioneered the belief that the physical body has the ability to hold emotional stress within the muscles and other body systems and imperial testing showed consistency of effects.

In 1949 Kendal and Kendall published a follow-up to the pioneer which further developed the art of the interconnectedness between body and mind.

Dr. Goodheart taught these processes and in further research linked chinese medicine, meridians and chiropractic techniques together which became known as Applied Kinesiology.

The 1970's saw Dr John Thie D.C. a student of Dr. Goodheart, develop 'Touch for Health', into a modality that allowed the public to begin to practice kinesiology at home.

WHY DO I NEED 'HOW TO: KINESIOLOGY?'

We all experience the ebb and flow of calmness and stress in our lives, be it physical, mental, emotional, spiritual or nutritional.

Kinesiology among other health modalities have known for a very long time that stress is the main cause of sickness. It's as if we get many reminders to look after ourselves and to not 'worry' about things that cannot be changed. Because of our humanness and our sense of self importance we often override what we know as our warning signs to slow down and take some attention to our bodies.

Yes, I totally understand that 'workplace, family and modern day needs' are important but so is our health and our ability to stay fully present in the moment. What tends to happen is our body reroutes itself to adapt, which in effect lessens our communication to our 'true' self. When this happens, it can affect all aspects of our psyche (physical, mental, emotional and spiritual).

The main type of kinesiology practiced at Bayside Kinesiology is HOW TO: Kinesiology? And Kinergetics, a dynamic and holistic approach which recognises that no two people are the same and aims to bring your body back into homeostasis or internally regulated equilibrium, giving you great understanding and leaving you feeling more in harmony with your environment.

Kinesiology is not a test of muscle strength, is not invasive, and does not require machines or complex diagnostic tools. It is an enlivening and enriching practice that helps us to understand others, and ourselves and often gives immediate answers to deep or unanswered and difficult questions that alternative medicines are unable to provide.

HOW DOES 'HOW TO: KINESIOLOGY?' WORK?

In HOW TO: Kinesiology? questions are asked of the client's body to find what area of stress is a priority to address. Kinesiology is used to help the body balance and restore communication.

Imagine for a moment if one type of stress is constantly repeated in many different ways during the course of your life how much of a mess you could very quickly get yourself into, in all honesty it can be as easy as shining truth on the cycle that happens.

- **Physical:**   I pulled a muscle while gardening

- Mental: My back is against the wall and I think that I am not good enough can cause strong back muscle tension

- **Emotional:**   I support the weight of the world on my shoulders

- **Spiritual:**   I am not following my spiritual path, allowing energy to flow through my spine

- Nutritional: I didn't drink enough water and my kidneys are not detoxifying properly

IF WE KNEW BETTER, WE WOULD DO BETTER - RIGHT?

HOW: TO Kinesiology? Helps us ask specific questions that result in greater understanding, self-awareness and health-giving energy.

ASK THE RIGHT QUESTIONS, GET THE RIGHT ANSWERS

HOW: TO Kinesiology? recognises that when emotions and exhaustion is high body intelligence is low. A kinesiologist simply asks the body which part needs improved communication and harmony. The body is designed to heal and grow, this happens when the body remains connected and communication pathways are able to work as a team. Believe it or not life is designed to be a win: win situation, it is our interpretation of events that get in the road and makes life difficult.

BACK TO WHOLENESS

Your body is designed to heal itself naturally. The physical body is the last to heal, when healing takes place in the energetic systems the physical has no other option other than to heal. Your whole body knows how to heal itself. It just needs to be reminded how.

HOW TO: KINESIOLOGY? DIFFERS FROM THE CONVENTIONAL HEALTH SYSTEM.

We take a holistic approach to health and happiness.

HOW TO: Kinesiology? identifies breakdowns of communication and asks the body for the priority and how it needs to heal in order to restore communication between all levels of the body.

Muscle test Video on YouTube: https://www.youtube.com/watch?v=kWJgnX-AhRQ

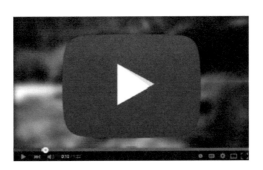

QUESTIONING SKILLS

The following are some examples of how to dig deeper in a treatment. The reason things come up for correction is because it is a stress for the body, but occasionally, we may need to muscle test to see if we need more or less of something.

- What would you do if you did know what to do?
- If it weren't such a big deal what would it be?
- Let's just get a 2% change. If that's easy to do, domino it to 4, 6, 8, 10%
- Don't sulk, yell, cry to avoid, it's not a get out of jail free card
- What is it you don't want to tell me/yourself?
- Do I need any more information here?
- If YES, **Physical**/Mental/**Emotional**/**Spiritual**/Nutritional? If NO, move on.
- For a deeper correction check 'in relation to the main issue does every (meridian) agree?
- Mythical creatures: Ask do I need more or less of this energy?
- What's the payoff for keeping this stress?
- Is it **Physical**/Mental/**Emotional**/**Spiritual**/Nutritional?

INTRODUCTION & ACKNOWLEDGEMENTS

Firstly, I need to say this book was hard. As a Kinesiologist I am passionate about what I do in the clinic, at my workshops and my retreats.

I hear your frustrations, Kinesiologists currently need only a measly 10 hours of managements skills for a certificate and a pathetic 25 hours for a diploma. It's no wonder so many amazing, beautiful, experienced therapists fail drastically even before they get off the ground.

So having said all that and after reading many, many sales, marketing and personal development books, listening to podcasts daily, webinars, videos, attending workshops, having private business management meetings, I still felt clueless on how to apply all this to the kinesiology world. I'm sure you're all nodding your heads!

It wasn't until I sat down and really pulled the business structure apart with a very dear, gifted, talented and amazing friend Kathy Mazlin, that I slowly started to get the 'ah ha' moments. I need to say right here and now that it still didn't come easily, as Kathy will agree to. But we have done it! I thank her for being strong with me and pushing me through the limitations that I created in my mind.

So now, my beautiful student and reader take solace in knowing I have done the hard work, chucked all the tantrums, had sleepless nights, budgeted and lost clinic hours for just you.

The good news is I realise that somewhere in the future you want to see a thriving business. I know you've got an internal image of yourself, of the impact you want to make in the world, and the people you want to serve. I know when you get to the end of your life and look back, you will wish that you had had the biggest impact with your kinesiology skills and that's exactly why I have put together this package of books plus course for you.

While at the point of production this book feels very comprehensive, it will always be incomplete, because technology is forever changing. Which is why I can't recommend highly enough to attend the 5-day workshop that complements this book.

This Abundance and Business Management course gives you

- Industry appropriate business skills - total saving of $3,500
- Kinesiology treatments - at least 2 per day saving over $1,500
- 5 days of holidays including fresh meals and accommodation at an additional ridiculously low price (we have had guests from around the world say it's been their best ever stay)
- Outdoor classroom amongst Australian wildlife (priceless)
- Airport pickup and drop offs – saving $150
- And
- I promise there will be no PowerPoint presentations or boring stuff!

OUR INDUSTRY SKILLS

We have so many beliefs surrounding healing work; some of them fit and others we need to let go and bury (see Appendix 6). One of the common beliefs is that most therapists are good at their art but not at paperwork, self-promotion, charging a sustainable amount and marketing... so let's clear all our negative programming on those things so we can bury that belief.

I absolutely know from experience how effective it is to clear our own negative programming in order to become better Kinesiologists. This manual in your hands is a testament to the effectiveness of the methods below.

Let's jump in, boots and all, and not judge what comes up for healing. It's important that if something comes up as a stress, you accept that somewhere, somehow IT IS a stress for you.

LET'S GET STARTED

We tend to be drawn to the energy and atmosphere of passionate people. If YOU love what YOU do, your enthusiasm, positivity, energy and excitement will serve to inspire, attract and engage your customers.

This means that instead of focusing on selling yourself, you will only have to educate your customers about your product or service and your passion will do the rest!

Get organised – so you have time to develop your passion. You need to be focused, passionate, driven, energetic, creative and strategic because you may have several positions to fulfil, such as: sales person, marketer, accountant, administrator, trouble shooter, techie, cleaner, secretary, teacher, counsellor, confidante, and 'gofer'. Not to mention often parent and spouse/partner as well!

Seek out mentors with relevant experience who will advise and help you achieve your success faster. Regular contact with your mentors will keep you on track. It also provides a great opportunity to brainstorm and share your ideas or challenges.

IT IS IN THE DNA

Every potential client has 3 basic behaviours: instinct, imagination and intelligence. Learn to market this simple formula.

Instinctual Behaviour

Breath rate, pulse rate, fight, flight mechanics, and reaction to environmental safety are automatic, instinctual behaviours. When marketing our aim is to not create doubt, fear, danger or suspicion in a customer's mind. Our brain filters through parameters. Viewers will switch off if fear, doubt, danger, complication, suspicion, boredom or uncertainty exists. Remember if it sounds too good to be true, it probably isn't true.

Imagination Behaviour

Imagination, vision, and future self all invoke imagination of what you want or do not want in the future. Understanding imagination behaviour needs to talk to the heart-centred vision of the customer. Where, in their heart, does the customer see themselves in 2 years? How does your product or service relate to that? We must appeal to their feelings, social meaning, dreams and emotional driven language.

Rational Intelligence

The processing, rational, thinking department of our brain decides if the service/product is a good return on investment, has good analysis, and provides facts and data. The customer must be able to trust you before they will invest.

SHADOW MARKETING

We all have a shadow side of fear, shame and guilt that we don't share with the world. At a very basic level everyone seeks:

- Attention
- To belong to something
- Control
- To be liked, superior or have a higher level of knowledge around a topic
- To be validated
- Money
- Sexuality – to be held, caressed, loved and cuddled

Marketing to the core drive of the human race of love, fear and guilt are the three fundamental building blocks of all marketing. By tailor marketing to one of these 7 core responses we link our future self to these core issues.

E.g. 1. Attention – love of, fear of, guilt of having...

KNOW YOUR CUSTOMERS

Index

Innovators (2.5%)

These are the consumers we need to be selling to, as they are the influencers. These people set the bar for healthy behaviour. They are:

- Trend setters, risk takers and early adopters
- Most health proactive
- Market leaders and influencers
- Users of some supplements
- Highest users of organic foods
- Users of many health modalities
- Most green
- Youngest in age
- Very social
- Financially savvy, having financial clarity

Early Adopters (13.5%)

These consumers represent a lucrative market that can be tapped into by providing the solutions and services they seek, primarily convenience and advice. They:

- Want to be healthy
- Are most likely to have children
- Are stressed out, want help and control
- Go on more health kicks but with no clear goal
- Are receptive to eco-friendly solutions
- Are actively into weight loss
- Are influential to other people
- Are also young in age
- Are slightly more discriminating in adoption choices than the innovators

Early Majority (35%)

These customers are seeking solutions to their health problems and are looking at every avenue. They are:

- "Conveniently healthy" only when it suits them
- Heavy pill users – supplement and prescription
- Health managers vs. preventers
- Weight managers
- Least likely to cook at home
- Least likely to exercise

Late Majority (34%)

These 'Food actives and Mainstream healthy conscious' are people going to the health food shops, looking for 'main stream convenience' answers to health issues. They:

- Have basic balance and control
- Desire inherently healthy foods
- Are most influenced by doctors
- Are least eco friendly
- Are price sensitive
- Are typically sceptical

Laggards (15%)

The most challenging segment to convert into sales in the natural health sector being that they are the most price sensitive and least eco-friendly. They are:

- Least health active
- Unconcerned about prevention
- Focused on taste
- Most price-driven
- Not concerned about weight loss
- Last to adopt an innovation
- Averse to change and prefer tradition

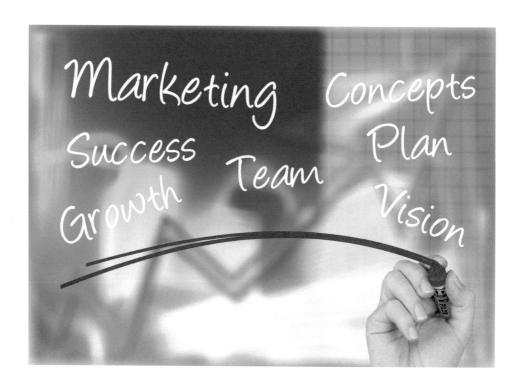

Where Are We Now?
"Situation Analysis"

Business Summary	Strengths & Weaknesses	Opportunities & Threats	Competitive Environment	My Competitive Advantages

Where Are We Going?
"Mission, Vision, Goals & Objectives"

Mission & Vision	Goals & Objectives

How Are We Going to Get There?
"Strategies & Action Plans"

Client Base	Marketing and Sales	Client Experience	Behind the Scenes

Review

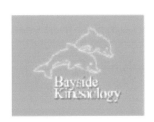

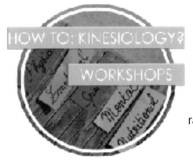

CONTACT

Bayside Kinesiology Brisbane,
Queensland AUSTRALIA

http://www.baysidekinesiology.com
ranee.zeller@baysidekinesiology.com

PH: 0419 737 396

THE BUSINESS PLANNING PROCESS

BUSINESS SUMMARY

Let's begin the planning process by developing a business summary for your business. It only needs to be one or two sentences. Below are some prompts to get you thinking.

Complementary medicine/therapies are a holistic approach to the prevention, and therapeutic management of a wide range of disorders within the community. We do not treat diseases or diagnose. Complementary medicine treats the cause and not the symptoms of any illness.

Because kinesiology is all about being holistic it is important to also follow this over into your business plan which is why we will be dissecting each of your business planning headings into the 5 sections of Physical, Mental, Emotional, Spiritual and Nutritional.

Physical

- How do you want to portray yourself physically within your business?
- What does your environment and clinic look like?
- Are you located in a good geographic area?
- Do you know key strengths/trends/impacts?
- Are the dollar investments and money returns working in your favour?
- What is your buying bargaining power? E.g. number of customer/size of each order/difference between/price sensitivity/ability to substitute/cost of changing
- What is your supplier power? E.g. number of suppliers/size of suppliers/uniqueness of service

Mental

- What type of client do you want to attract to you?
- Are you mentally 100% with your clients for the duration of their visit?

Emotional

- What is the emotional investment you have in your clients getting better or returning?
- Does your personal reputation depend on your professional successes?
- How do you want your client to feel after the first treatment?
- What is your emotional guarantee you can offer to your client immediately?
- Is your 'heart' in your business?
- Does being in this industry bring you joy?

Spiritual

- Are you a spiritual therapist, if so, what are your beliefs and boundaries here?
- Do you offer spiritual advice?
- Do you feel that you are attracting the type of spiritual guidance and support that you need for yourself and your clients?
- Do you have any 'rituals' that you do before the day or between each client?

Nutritional

- Are you going to offer nutritional advice?
- Do you walk your talk in relation to your personal nutrition?
- Do you have a support system of other nutritional specialist referrals to fill in the gaps of your nutritional knowledge?

STRENGTHS

Next, we will look at where your business is right now. Think about what its strengths and weaknesses are. Again, I have set out some questions to help you look at your business objectively. Work through them and see which ones resonate for you.

Strengths are positive attributes, tangible and intangible, internal to your organisation within your control.

Physical

- Do you have and adhere to appropriate codes of conduct (see Appendix 3 for examples)
- What do you do well?
- What internal resources do you have?
- What are the positive attributes of yourself/team? E.g. knowledge, background, education, credentials, network, reputation, or specific skills
- What are your tangible assets? E.g. capital, credit, existing customers or distribution channels, patents, or technology
- Does the design of building/facility/studio reflect your environmental beliefs?
- Is the clinic in a good geographic location for clients/transport/advertising?
- Are you visible in the community offering excellent public goodwill?
- Do you/your team offer excellent service both in application and referral?
- Are your services and technical appliances up to date in relation to current trends?
- Are your services/products ethically sourced and priced?
- Do you contribute back to the community? E.g. in dollars or time
- Is your team dedicated, what are the unique 'in house' points? E.g. flexible hours: the time it takes to do vs. the hours you have to be at work?
- Have your business goal deadlines been set into a business calendar so you know when to action them?
- Are your business goals clearly prioritised and on display?
- Are there rewards for success/progress for self/team?
- Is accountability clearly defined? E.g. are you/your team empowered to seek help from mentors and team to break tasks down into do-able action steps
- Has the business automated as much as possible? E.g. bills/promotions/passive income/customer booking system
- Do you know what business goal came true for the last financial year?
- Based on past positive feedback, have you actioned what experiences the business wants to have reoccur over the next 4/6/12 months?
- Can you be clear on financial goals to be achieved in the next 4/6/12 months?
- Do you strategise? E.g. mailing list/social media followings to grow 200% over 12 months?

Mental

- Do you know your unique brand positioning?
- What internal advantages do you have over your competition?
- How do you add value or offer differently to your competitors?
- Do you have strong research and development capabilities?
- Are you known for good clinical outcomes?
- Do you have accountability on challenges/positive outcomes with customers/team service previous 4/6/12 month periods?
- How do you make a conscious effort to learn from the lessons/challenges you had when working with your team/suppliers/public?
- Do you have a record of gross profit for the last 4/6/12 month period? (Total amount of dollars that came into your business)
- Can you access records of total expenses for the last 4/6/12 month period?
- Do you have a record of net profit for the previous 4/6/12 month period? (Total income less expenses)
- Can you access records of top five sellers/products during last period?
- Can you access records of how much in dollar value they earned?
- Do you review/action/repeat the biggest highlights of the last 12 months?
- Do you review/action/repeat what's working in the business right now? E.g. marketing strategies/product/service/processes
- Do you invest in programs/resources/lectures/self-development courses?
- Do you know how much time/money/health/support/communication is needed to set aside to be able to complete this education in the next 4/6/12 month period?
- Do you review/action what didn't work so well? E.g. systems/automations/working to long hours/customers service/publicity or supplier
- Do you review business mission/vision statement?
- Do you know how big the mailing list is, and how much it increased over the last 4/6/12 month period?
- Do you know how many social media followers your business currently has? E.g. Facebook/Twitter/Instagram/LinkedIn/Periscope and how much it increased over the last 12-month period?
- Do you know what marketing worked this 4/6/12 month period and why it worked?
- Do you know your ideal customers in detail? Can you accurately market to them? E.g. age/gender/experiences/outcomes

Emotional

- Do you understand clients' needs, wants, and behaviours?
- Do you understand client's identification? E.g. medical/sexual/religious
- Have you built up a commendable history and reputation?
- Do you and your team show caring, competent and clinical professionalism?
- Can your word be relied upon?
- Do you celebrate your new products/announcements?
- Have you a good work/life balance?
- Do you know in detail what a perfect 'work' day looks like?
- Do you have clarity on what clientele the business wants to attract? E.g. family/partnerships/corporate clientele
- Do you know how self/staff make an impact in people's life?
- Have you scheduled in holidays for self/team?

Spiritual

- Does your business offer a comprehensive service with a holistic approach?
- Does the way you deliver your services align with your spiritual beliefs? Integrity, ethics, religious E.g. laws of karma, not work on Sundays...
- Do you give back to the world/community or cause money/time/donation of services/products?
- Do you write and review gratitude diary of all the amazing things that have gone well for you in business and personal life?
- Do you set goals in different key areas of personal and business life so as to continually fuel your goals?

Nutritional

- Do you support your local, ethical 'farmacy'?
- Are your products of optimal nutritional worth?
- Do you have clarity on your own health and wellbeing goals, as they will impact on business life?

WEAKNESSES

Weaknesses are factors that are within your control that detract from your ability to obtain or maintain a competitive edge?

Physical

- Do you have mentors you can turn to in all areas of business? Are you using their skills actively enough? If you could choose any mentor, who would it be? E.g. financial/marketing/graphics/editor/spiritual/nutritional or emotional
- What is keeping you from growing your team? E.g. skill set, time, money or suppliers
- What areas need improvement to accomplish your objectives or compete with your strongest competitor?
- Is your clinic/business in a poor location?
- Does your clinic/business have a high staff turnover?
- Do you have to be master of every area of your business? E.g. Therapist/book keeper/cleaner/marketer?
- Is English the only spoken language?
- Do you have poor market preparation/positioning?
- Is there low true value in what you are offering?
- Does your business have poor follow up procedures?
- Are your products appropriately/safely stored?
- Do you have a clean working environment?
- Do your premises meet all safety standards?
- Are you/your business in a poor position of making business decisions? E.g. franchise obligations, modality restrictions?
- Is the dress code/personal appearance poor?
- Is the stamina of yourself/your team physically poor?
- Do your premises need a physical spring clean?
- Do you need to enrol into a course to enhance/refresh/learn new skills?
- Do you have standard operation procedures to provide a starting point and save valuable time? Is everyone aware of them and how they function? E.g. business correspondence: font/margins/header/footer/emails/signatures

- Are there policy procedures in place for bookings/cancelations/refunds?
- What are the responsibilities for self/staff? E.g. facilities/marketing/ordering and financials, and are they operating effectively?
- Is your accounting system able to do all that is needed? E.g. access to statistics on income/expenses/taxes/products/services
- Are financials prepared on time and ready to be audited?

Mental

- What do you perceive your competitive weaknesses are?
- Does your clinic lack expertise or access to skills or technology?
- Does your business have limited resources?
- Do you lack social media competency?
- Do you lack computer skills?
- Are you unsure of the focus for the business this year?
- What are your coping mechanisms when things get too hard?
- Are you unsure where to find relevant programs/resources/lectures to give you the skills you need to invest in?
- Are you unsure how much time you/your staff need to set aside to be able to complete education?

Emotional

- Do you have your own professional support system when you get difficult clients?
- How do you switch off the 'connection' after a client leaves?
- Do you have strong healthy emotional boundaries?
- What is the emotional investment you have attached to outcomes?
- Do you lack consistency/motivation?
- Do you feel like there are not enough hours in the day for you to be successful in all areas of your business?
- What is your internal communication with other staff or yourself?
- Do you focus too much on the future without celebrating past successes? E.g. for the week/business/clients/team
- Do you feel confident the business could run smoothly if you are away from it for any amount of time?
- Do you know the homework that is needed for the lessons learnt? E.g. write down your thoughts or have a kinesiology session. Can you release in order to let go and start afresh or apologise?
- Have you set achievable goals for yourself/team? Perfection is a perception, not a reality as perception is always changing

Spiritual

- What is your known spiritual practice that will assist you to get back into balance when you fall?
- Where are your business practices out of alignment with your spiritual beliefs?
- Do your premises need an energy clean?
- Are there inconsistent cultural images in your business practice? E.g. Christian symbols, Buddha statues or professional image vs. casual image

Nutritional

- What are your food weaknesses when you feel out of alignment? Decide before this happens how you will auto correct them before they cascade into disaster

OPPORTUNITIES

In the next two sections we will look at what you can foresee happening for your business in the near future that you may need to factor into your plans. These are the "opportunities" and "threats" to your business.

Opportunities are positive, attractive factors that represent reasons your business is likely to prosper.

Physical

- What do you need to be the best version of yourself, to thrive as a manager over the next year? E.g. social time/mindful meditation/fitness/family and friend support/leisure and travel/learning and development
- In what ways can your business create a better world? Recycle/reduce/reuse/social and environmental performance accountability/transparency
- What opportunities exist in your market or the environment that you can benefit from?
- Can you improve your physical environment considering the 5 senses? Add music, change colour scheme, burns oils, warm towels…
- Has there been a recent market growth or have there been other changes in the market that have created an opportunity?
- Is the opportunity ongoing, or is there just a window of time to act? How critical is your timing?
- Do you support customer loyalty? How?
- Is there an unsaturated market, which can tolerate the opening of a new practice/product?
- Can you secure affiliation with other centres/groups/professionals to enhance your reputation and referral network?
- How strong are your rehabilitation/after services to wellness business models?
- Healthcare policy makers are pursuing cost saving measures, how can you make this in your favour?
- Do you offer real and effective solutions in an expansive range of health settings?
- Are there government or charitable group that you can align with? E.g. community support groups/ grants/ funding opportunities
- Can you design and offer client handouts on a range of subjects? Do you know what business skill you want to develop over the next 4/6/12 months? E.g. seminars/ marketing/ spiritual

Mental

- Can the perception of your business be improved?
- Can you increase involvement in policy making under branch associations?
- What is the next foreseeable change in market trend?
- How effective are your virtual events? Do you deliver them often enough? Do you market them well?
- Do you offer eLearning?

Emotional

- Do you offer real and effective emotional support settings via community/one-on-one/audio?
- Can you improve the emotional engagement of clients by increasing their comfort within your treatment environment? How/where are you going to get the necessary help to achieve this?
- Can you create a vision board of all the possible and impossible (there is no such word as impossible, it actually says I'm possible) goals to achieve if anything was possible this 4/6/12 month period? Know who would be with you/where you would go/what you would do
- Are there self-care rules in place in order to keep sane at work?
- Are you able to forgive yourself? Can you review goals, talk to a friend, meditate, reflect, stop, look and listen to outside help?
- Do you have a clean working environment? How can you/your team embrace the business culture?

Spiritual

- Can you offer an understanding and possible network where clients can connect to their own spiritual principles for comfort/guidance and support?

Nutritional

- Can you refer and recommend individual nutritional programs, whether you are qualified to do this yourself or do you outsource?
- Can you do a monthly bulk order for your clients?
- Do you offer healthy recipes to get people started?
- Can you run workshops for cooking? E.g. lunchbox/gluten free/vegetarian/athletic/elderly

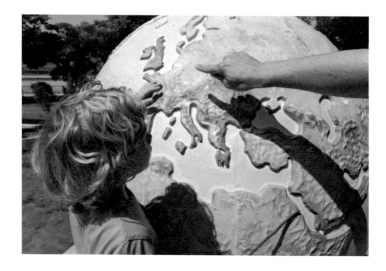

THREATS

Threats include external negative factors beyond your control that could place your strategy, or the business itself, at risk.

You have no control over these, but you may benefit by having contingency plans to address them if they should occur.

Physical

- Are existing or potential competitors encroaching on your business territory?
- Has there been a significant change in supplier prices or the availability of raw products?
- Has a new product or technology been introduced that makes your products, equipment, or services obsolete?
- Are the healthcare authorities changing policies in a way that changes your business practices? E.g. health rebates/policy changes

Mental

- Are there challenges created by an unfavourable trend or development that may lead to deteriorating revenues or profits?
- What situations might threaten your marketing efforts?
- Has there been a shift in the economy or government regulations that could reduce your sales?
- Are there legal battles over scope of practice?
- Are you focussing too much on the clinical delivery of your services, and not enough on business/law/politics and policies?
- Is your ego bruised when the responsibilities of yourself/your staff regarding facilities/marketing/ordering/financials change or when 'new blood' comes into your business?
- Do you know that the business will provide a pay each week?

Emotional

- Has there been a shift in consumer behaviour that could reduce your sales?
- Is there burn out in your professional culture?

Spiritual

- Is there professional competition within your practice driven from the ego?
- Do your business premises give off a 'bad vibe'?
- Is your pride and authority in your profession being ruled by the ego or external perceived competition?

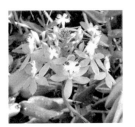

Nutritional

- Are there bigger companies stamping out the smaller farmers locally?
- If you/your team are unsure of a nutritional product, will you still recommend it because there is a dollar in it for you?

COMPETITIVE ENVIRONMENT

The competitive environment is the external environment of your industry E.g. other therapists, facilities, modalities, marketing strategies.

At this part of the planning process it is important to look at who the competitors to your business are so you can be ready to respond as your competitive environment changes.

Physical

- Do you know who your major competitors are that will directly affect your business? E.g. who is competing for the same target clientele?
- What is the number of competitors that influence your trade locally/globally?
- How well do you know what your competitor's objectives and resources are?
- Do your competitors have a more competitive pricing structure? E.g. are they more compassionate to: pensioners/unemployed/children
- Are your competitors keeping up with trends faster than you are?
- Do you have new niche competitors? How easy are you to copy?
- Do you strongly know your competitors' business offerings/size/tactics skill set?
- What are the quality differences in services/product/resources/support between you and your competitors?
- Is your business placed in a better demographic area than your competitors?
- Do your competitors have more up-to-date business technologies?

Mental

- Do you regularly review your competitive marketing strategies?
- Will you be surprised by the threat of substitute goods/services?
- Is there internal rivalry within your industry? Do you work with this in a positive or negative way?

Emotional

- In comparison to your competitors, do you over-deliver/under-deliver for your customers' emotional needs? E.g. furnishings/colour of interior/ambient lighting/outdoor environment/comfort food
- Do your competitors offer a better customer loyalty program than your business?

Spiritual

- Do you offer spiritual workshops/mediation at more favourable times for your clients than your competitors have?
- Do you offer better information services than your competitors? E.g. books/handouts/visuals/YouTube/awakened documentaries

Nutritional

- What are your competitors doing in the nutritional area? E.g. can you offer/recommend local organic/fair trade products/producers?

COMPETITIVE ADVANTAGE/POINT OF DIFFERENCE

Your unique selling proposition (USP) is the marketing statement you use to sell your products and services to a prospective customer.

Develop a catchy easy to remember sales slogan, focusing on your customer's needs and wants.

Your competitive advantage is what sets your business apart from your competition. It highlights the benefits a customer receives when they do business with you. It could be your products, service, reputation, or even your location.

In order to get your message across effectively you have to market yourself by addressing the 'why', 'what', and 'how' in that order.

Questions to ask:

Why

- Why do customers buy from us?
- Why do customers buy from our competitors and not us?
- Why do some potential customers not buy at all?
- Identify clients 'pain point'. What is a problem to them?
- Acknowledge their pain point within the first 30 seconds of interaction; otherwise the sale is likely to be lost
- Why do they need to come to you? Make it easy for them to understand why their life/career/relationships/abundance/weight/learning issue needs your product or service

What

- What does the customer want?
- What need or want are they really trying to satisfy?
- What is the main reason my customers buy from me?
- What can I do to match or exceed those expectations?
- What can I do to make sure the customer gets what they want?
- What's involved?
- What's included?
- What will it look like?

How

- Although it can be difficult to explain exactly how kinesiology works, providing examples of success stories will demonstrate that it works!
- Simple explanations can also be found on the websites of kinesiology associations
- How can my uniqueness be made different from my competitors?

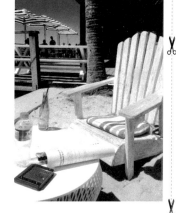

Physical

- Make life simpler?
- Operate at more flexible times than your competitors to support your customer's family/childcare situations?
- Reflect excellence of quality?
- Reflect is your business preferable, but not necessarily unique?
- Maintain advertising freshness and viability?
- Change over time as competitors try to cash in on your trends?
- Reflect good "bang for your buck"?
- Provide excellent services/skill sets?
- Provide clean and safe facilities?
- Provide a wide choice of availability of quality/quantity or variety?
- Have more than one unique offer? If you only have one unique offer people may be able to copy it, if you have two it makes for a stronger brand

Mental

- Focus on one product/service as a specialty?
- "Fix" a problem, therefore possibly being able to charge more for your knowledge/expertise?
- Market to your customer's needs better than your competitors? E.g. time and money constraints?
- Provide clear and simple solutions?

Emotional

- Help clients feel better about themselves?
- Know what the clientele wants and needs emotionally? E.g. how is your bedside manner?
- Present newsworthy information?
- Support honest and ongoing market research?
- Highlight the benefits to customers?
- Have better public visibility than your competitors? E.g. social media/TV/magazines/radio

Spiritual

- Offer spiritual leanings: retreats/chanting/singing bowls/yoga/tai chi?

Nutritional

- Have its own herbal tea blend/something else unique to your region/clinic?
- Have a signature aromatherapy blend that people connect to you/clinic when they smell it? Where are you going?

Congratulations

You have now done the hard work of being totally honest with where your business "sits" right now. In management speak you have done your situation analysis.

Now it's time to have fun with your business vision, the driver, motivator and reason for being in business. The reason to start planning is so you can turn your dreams into reality....
Lets' get started, it's your time to shine and dream big.

What do you want? Why are you in business?

See Appendix 2 for some examples of famous statements

WHERE ARE WE GOING?

MISSION AND VISION

Mission Statement

Identities values and purposes of a business that is formally written to show the business set of ethos.

It is a simple statement of: "Who we are and what we do".

Vision Statement

A Vision Statement is a sentence or short paragraph providing a broad, inspirational image of the future. A Vision statement is defined as 'An Image of the future we seek to create'.

Combine physical, emotional, and logical elements into one exceptional customer and employee experience.

My vision for the business is: I/my team/my business will have/be (insert relevant descriptive words below) therapy clinic in (geographic location).

Business Planning

Physical

- Backbone
- Braver
- Conquer
- Diverse
- Physical
- Stunning
- Valour

- Biggest
- Breath taking
- Courage
- Epic
- Sensational
- Technologically advanced
- Vanquish

- Bold
- Cheerful
- Daring
- Legendary
- Spectacular
- Triumph
- Victory

Mental

- Accredited
- Attached
- Best-selling
- Certified
- Excellence
- Fully refundable
- Innovative
- Leadership
- No obligation
- No strings attached
- Privacy protected
- Recession-proof
- Research
- Solution orientated
- There is always a way
- Unconditional
- Well respected

- Anonymous
- Authentic
- Cancel anytime
- Different
- Flexibility
- Guaranteed
- Integrity
- Lifetime
- No questions asked
- Official
- Proven
- Recognized
- Results
- Team orientated
- Track record
- Variety

- Approved
- Backed
- Case-study reliable
- Endorsed
- Freedom
- Income
- Knowledge
- Money-back
- No risk
- Open-minded
- Receptive
- Refund
- Secure
- Tested
- Try before you buy
- Verify

Emotional

- Bold
- Cheerful
- Excited
- Grateful
- Heartfelt
- Hope
- Jubilant
- Remarkable
- Trust
- Bravery
- Courageous
- Eye-opening
- Gutsy
- Heroic
- Intimate
- Mind-blowing
- Staggering
- Wonderful
- Breath taking
- Creative
- Fearless
- Happy
- Honesty
- Jaw-dropping
- Miracle
- Surprising

Spiritual

- Angelic
- Belief
- Conquer
- Devoted
- Evolve
- Genuine
- Innocent
- Mind-blowing
- Religious
- Ripple effect
- Spirit
- True
- Authenticity
- Blissful
- Constant
- Enchant
- Faith
- Godly
- Loyal
- Miracle
- Respectful
- Sensational
- Steadfast
- Virtuous
- Awe-inspiring
- Celebrate
- Dedicated
- Eye-opening
- Faithful
- Good
- Magic
- Pure
- Reverent
- Spectacular
- Super-human
- Wondrous

Nutritional

- Acidic
- Crisp
- Flavourful
- Full-bodied
- Infused
- Light
- Refreshing
- Robust
- Aged
- Earthy
- Fresh
- Hearty
- Juicy
- Medicinal
- Rich
- Tender
- Alkaline
- Fermented
- Fruity
- Herbal
- Lean
- Raw
- Ripe
- Zesty

GOALS & OBJECTIVES

Now that you know where your business really is having done your situation analysis (past and present) and you have done your creative "visioning" of where your business is going, you can now set realistic business goals for the future (next 4/6/12 months)
They must be quantifiable and measurable.

The components of your business that you will be setting your goals for fall into the following 4 categories.

- Client base: e.g. adults, children, animals, students, corporates
- Marketing and sales: How the client got there
- Customer Experience: what the customer sees and experiences:
- Product and   service delivery facilities and studios E.g. each modality, books, workshops, clinic rooms, ambience
- Behind the scenes – All support systems E.g. Finance, accounting, management and organisational systems. E.g. emails, client data basis, files, associations, continual professional education, first aid…

Prioritise your top 7-10 goals for this financial year, (having too many major goals scatters your energies too thin and can become too hard to achieve).

Once the 7-10 goals are chosen – what goals actions do you need to take in order for them to systemise onto a calendar so you can't fail?

Are your goals S.M.A.R.T? Specific, measurable, actionable, realistic, time-bound. Whatever the goal, small daily investments can bring you big results.

People tend to overestimate what they can do in a week and under estimate what they can achieve in a year.

Here are some examples below to get you thinking of the types of goals that could help your business soar to the next level:

Client Base

- I will increase my client base by 20% this financial year
- I will expand my client base to include more children visits by 10%
- I will ensure that I increase my clients repeat visits by...
- I will conduct a client survey in January asking: How could we improve your experience? With these answers I will make appropriate changes by February

Marketing and Sales

- I will have a social media and trade show presence by the end of August
- I will write a monthly BLOG starting from January
- I will spend $600 on updating my webpage
- I will update my web page by February to include the new modality I am offering
- I will spend $x on Facebook to improve the visibility of my courses
- I will run stalls at 2 trade fairs/expos this financial year
- I will run a trade stand at an expo to be held in Toowoomba in March
- This financial year I will place 5 advertisements in Mothers' magazines
- I will promote my services on all association webpages
- I will do a radio interview/podcast before Christmas to advertise my holiday specials

Customer Experiences

- I will expand my knowledge of anatomy and be able to name and show the range of motion for the 16 main muscles used in kinesiology by March
- I will produce and have client handouts available for celiac, dairy and nut allergies by February
- I will revamp my clinic room with a new colour scheme and purchase Christmas oils for December
- I will make a herb garden at the front of the studio front entrance by September

Behind the Scenes

- I will buy a new massage table before October
- I will update my accounting system before 30/6
- I will automate my patient record system by April
- I will update my mailing list by June 30th
- I will introduce Reiki to my practice by November
- I will publish my latest book in January
- I will run my Kinesiology workshop in September
- I will automate my known bills E.g. associations, insurances, memberships

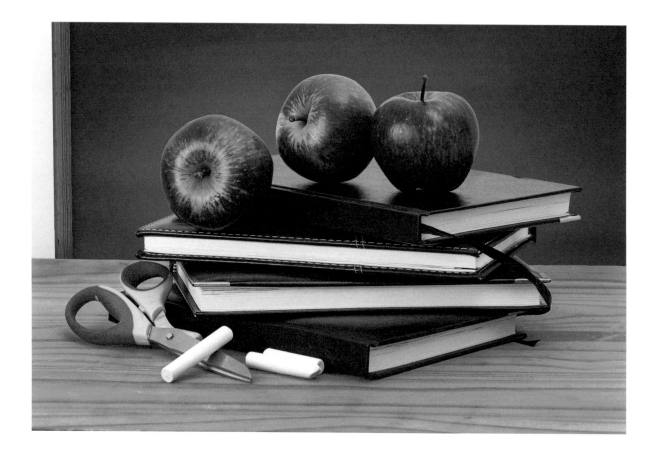

HOW ARE WE GOING TO GET THERE? STRATEGIES & ACTION PLAN

So now it's time to develop the goals that are your highest priority for the business. Here are some prompts to help you to design/flesh out your action items on your goals. Once you have your 7 – 10 goals then do bullet points specifically to each goal in each area (client base, marketing and sales, customer experience, behind the scenes).

CLIENT BASE

Physical

- Can you have a TV in your waiting room promoting services?
- What do you need to do to have 20 clients per week?
- How can you nurture "family" type of clients?

Mental

Where you can offer your skill set:

- Financial groups
- Education and personal development groups
- Fitness groups
- Health seekers
- Home improvers audience
- Lifestyle/adrenalin seekers
- Rehabilitation groups
- Retirement groups
- Spiritual development groups
- Travellers
- Weight management support

Emotional

- How can you clearly and concisely connect the client emotionally with their goal for each treatment?
- How do you look after your clients on an emotional level, what sort of personal information do you keep on file about them?

Spiritual

- What direction can you take yourself/your business that is authentic to your branding/style of service? Expos/lectures/dances/Feng Shui/meditation
- How can you always aim to clear your own/clients negative spiritual attachments?

Nutritional

- How can you stay with a clear purpose of the benefits of changing lifestyle dietary intakes? Do you have the right language to portray this importance?
- How can you/your business express themselves creatively? What would it feel like? E.g. soft, caring, strong, informative, formal
- What creative direction can you give for nutrition? E.g. food foraging classes/make & bake/raw food/fermentation/gluten education

MARKETING & SALES

Physical

- How much net income per week do you want your business to be worth?
- How can you announce points of interest on answering machine while people are waiting to be attended to?
- How do you set innovative goals to find new ways to improve? E.g. products/services/how you market your business/how you distribute and deliver what your business sells?
- What are the profitability goals/sights on where you want your bottom line to be for the next 4/6/12 months?
- How do you expand the creative ownership over your business? E.g. design/ branding/ facility?
- How can you reinvent your product/service/technique/process to stay ahead of the trend? E.g. go beyond servicing basic needs
- How can you make your product/service/technique/process remarkable enough/simple to explain/easy to demonstrate that people will drive across the country just for you? Will they take the time to learn about your product/service?
- How can you make your slogan catchy/matching the business perception?
- Can you make it easy for people to remember or is it spreadable? E.g. McDonalds- golden arches, Toyota – oh what a feeling, Nike – just do it, Bayside Kinesiology – love this life
- Have you targeted your advertising to be cost effective? Don't try to please everyone, better to be a big fish in a small pond than a small fish in a large pond
- How are you going to reward the clients that love you? www.sethgodwin.com is a legend for marketing and promotional ideas
- Is this trend/way of marketing got a time line on it? Do you need to act fast to catch the market? E.g. festive occasions promotions/responding to a major global disaster/birth of someone's new idea that you can piggyback on? E.g. new drug found to help with dieting vs. you can clear the cause and not just treat the symptom
- How can you make a collection/package version of your product/service? E.g. discount for full moon clients/buy the complete set and get one free
- Can you bring back a classic idea? E.g. offer an overhaul treatment for the new seasons with nothing specific to treat/stay ahead of your health/better to pay to stay healthy than pay to repair
- How can you "pull the pin" on an idea and start again? Do you set yourself up with a budget or time frame prior to launching?
- How can you launch a product/service that competes with yourself? E.g. selling a book that has all the information vs. you will get more from doing a workshop
- How can you learn from failure? Failure is not the opposite of success it's part of success, F.A.I.L = First Attempt In Learning, the only true failure is when you stop trying
- How can you make a list of ways you could catch-up by being different, acknowledging that you will never catch-up by being the same?
- What steps could you take to give your marketing budget for the next 4/6/12 months to a designer to get fresh ideas?
- Can you create a marketing environment where you can invent a new trend in time to replace the last one when it inevitably trails off?
- How can you package your product incredibly? Sometimes it's not the product but the packaging that sells. E.g. being seen at a luxurious day spa = stress elimination, holidaying at the mountain in a tent = recharging, computer gadgets = de-cluttering or systemising

- How can you modify your product/service so that you show up in the next trade magazine/be on Dr Phil/wherever your goal to be is?
- Can you do an honour system where people pay you what they can afford or what they think your worth? This can also be inviting someone to pay for the next clients treatment showing an act of kindness or by paying it forward
- How can you get permission from your previous clients to alert them via email of your promotions?
- What percentage will you spend on expenses in your business in the next budgeting period? E.g. purchasing assets/liabilities/cost of sales/expenses
- How can your service/product match your business brand? E.g. selection/ features/ pricing/ service?
- How can you become more aware, some people need up to ten touch points before they commit? E.g. we have something planned for you, it involves…., or little gold nuggets of what they will learn at the event
- How can you get to know your ideal customer in detail so that you can accurately market to them? E.g. age/gender/experiences
- Could you run a customer survey? What would make the business a better experience? E.g. what do you like/dislike about our business? What is one thing we could improve on? What is your biggest frustration about our product/service? What do you like most about our product/service?
- Can you survey your customers to see where they need the most help? E.g. family/relationships/leisure/travel/financial/legal/health/lifestyle/paid work/non-paid work/life-long learning and development
- How can the business reward loyal customers practically and emotionally? E.g. free stuff/discounts/information nights/celebration occasions evening
- How can the business capture client testimonials/referrals?
- What free opt-in offers will you create this next 4/6/12 month period that will entice people to sign up and follow your business? Free products/services samples/guides/weekly tips/recipes for success/product reviews?
- How can you provide expert advice and professionalism/bundling and packaging/ adding different levels of service based upon client's frequency or amount of purchase/frequent buyer programs?
- How can you educate customers to be able to utilise the products?
- How can you improve speed of service or delivery?
- How can you keep customer up to date with latest research?
- Where do you want to be seen promoting? E.g. local paper/billboards/festival/ podcasts/periscope/school newsletters/speaking gigs/networking events
- What new trends/products/services/blog posts/newspaper articles will you aim to create this next 4/6/12 month period?
- How can you source/purchase local/ethical products?
- How can you deliver what you say you will?
- How can you improve on the business distribution and order handling proficiency?
- How can you have a business that 'matches your ethos' distributing your products?
- When purchasing/invoicing can you add a personalised/quirky thank you for your prompt attention gimmick? E.g. chocolate/letter/tip
- How can you up-sell? E.g. discounts/promotions/relevant information from affiliated businesses?
- Can you offer promotional items? Do they need to be manufactured/produced? Do you have convenient storage space for them?

- Can you run more than one webinar/workshop/event because they will gain momentum?
- Can you offer a 'bring a friend for free'/'half price strategy' to bring more people through your doors, as it makes the person think about who is one person I can bring?
- How can you publish small teasers of what's coming up via social media and your database as you get closer to the event to which will re-awaken their interest?
- Can you run a competition depending on how long your promotional time frame is? E.g. to enter you need to do... to receive a free entry ticket. Use social media so people share your event with friends
- Can you do more social media: Facebook/ LinkedIn/ Twitter/ Instagram/ Podcast/ own radio station
- Can you do more mail outs: snail mail/newsletters/press releases/thank you notes/client worksheets & homework?
- Do you have a web opt-in page?
- Where can you advertise your: Webinar/workshop/event/blogs/conference
- Where can you be seen publicly at E.g. trade shows/festivals
- Where can you advertise in: magazine articles/community notice/ online magazines boards/coupons/back of shopper docket/Google ads/sponsorships/YouTube advertisements?
- Can you revamp your web/brochures/business cards/email signature/envelopes or external packaging/flyers/name tags/office or design space signage/office stationary with business name or logo?
- Can you advertise on: public transport/shopping carts/points of purchase/your own vehicle?
- Can you become an affiliate or member/key note speaker/presenter/M.C?
- How can you create a partnership so everyone has a win: win where you reward a partner by giving them money for selling your tickets or you help to also promote them at the same time as yourself? E.g. you are allowed to have a stand at their event
- Can you join a networking group/event in order to meet and talk to others where you can also invite them to come to your event?
- Can you send out something promotional that is amazing so it stands out via direct mail?
- Can you create a product/service where kids tell parents then parents tell others?

Mental

- How can you keep your regular customers rather than need to find a new client?
- How do you retain clear emotional objectives of why you work?
- How are you unique to all the other businesses in your field? Why your business/product/service?
- Can you increase brand awareness?
- How can you invite the client to change their behaviour to make your business more streamline? E.g. teach them to book an appointment on line?
- Can your product/service/technique/process be remarkable enough/simple to explain/easy to demonstrate that people will drive across the country just for you? Will they take the time to learn about your product/service?
- Do you know how tightly knit your target market is? How can you get them to talk about you openly? Will they spread the word for you? Do they believe each other?
- How can you differentiate your customers to find the group that is more profitable/decisive? E.g. loyal clients/students
- Can you redefine what you sell? Language is constantly changing; stay young and fresh in your approach

- Can you copy from another industry? E.g. Apple computers sell: more capable/versatile/portable/compatible, they don't display technical information on storage capacity/size/weight/chip size until much later. They recognise most of their customers don't care. Don't oversell the technical in your business either
- Have you made a list of remarkable products/services in your industry? Do you know who made them and why? Can you mimic the behaviour (not the product)?
- Can you upgrade your accounting system you use? E.g. Ease/portable/comprehensive/delivers reports/charts/sends reminders/tracks
- Can you update relevant current competitor analysis?
- Do you know your customer requirements? E.g. physically/mentally/emotionally/nutritionally/spiritually
- Where can you source your market information statistics?
- Do you know who/where to find your potential customer?
- Can your staff stay up to date with your products/services? Do you offer regular sales training/planning?
- Can you remarket by showing contents/adds/teasers/ to people that have already visited your events page?
- Can you Google advertise more effectively?
- Can you do affiliate marketing, where you partner up with people who have a great database with a similar audience? (Affiliates get a certain amount of each ticket price they sell)

Emotional

- How can you offer a solution for people who are feeling emotional/vulnerable and are very influenced to external marketing messages?
- Do you know where the product/service ends and the perception/hype begins? E.g. bedside manner/weirdness or uniqueness can be marketed/setting or location/environmental factors
- Can you differentiate criticism of a product/service vs. taking things personally? The key to failure is trying to please everyone all of the time
- How are you going to reward the clients that love you?
- What improvements can you make to your business? Brand, identity, or personality? E.g. consistency/provide excellent customer service/builds a community/make a difference/treat every client like a VIP
- Can you find an angle for your clinic/workshop/event/webinar to be irresistible?
- Are you marketing towards the needs of your business? Is it organically emotionally based? What percentage?
- Do you know what makes you unique to all the other businesses in your field? Why your business/product/service?
- Can you offer a money back guarantee? Most people feel warm and fuzzy when offered this, but very few follow through on claims
- Can you market to the customers' emotions? The longer the waiting list the more emotionally important things seem to get

Spiritual

- How are you marketing the spiritual aspect of your business?
- What new trends/products/services/blog posts/newspaper articles will you create this 4/6/12 month period?

Nutritional

- Can your business have a shop front for supplements/powders
- Can you sell gadgets that make healthy eating easy? E.g. grain sprouting equipment/dehydrator/Thermomix

CUSTOMER EXPERIENCE

This is what the customer sees and experiences: Product and service delivery facilities and studios E.g. each modality, books, workshops, clinic rooms.

Physical

- Can your facilities/studio be big enough to grow into?
- Can the business have enough car parking e.g. time limit on parking/easy for handicap people if the business grows?
- How can you provide easy access to clinic from road/handicap people to access all parts of the facilities?
- Can you display the licensing and permits appropriate?
- How will you meet health standards?
- Do you have adequate business building and content insurance?

Emotional

- How do you want the space to be perceived? E.g. professional/warming/family orientated/safe/professional/up market/elite
- How can you enhance the kinaesthetic of the environment? E.g. pets for therapy/garden area/smell/visuals/comfort
- How does the team have brainstorming sessions? Can you generate questions that enhance ideas?

Spiritual

- Can your facility be colourful like the chakras or white reflecting enlightenment?
- Can you do an energy clearing on the space/location/offices?
- Can you have Feng Shui symbols around to enhance energy flow?
- How can your business display spirituality? Does eastern culture deter other religions? E.g. Christians

BEHIND THE SCENES

- Behind the scenes is where you have all your support systems of finance, accounting, management and organisational systems E.g. emails, client data base, files, associations, continual professional education, first aid.

Physical

- Can you generate questions that enhance brainstorming sessions?
- Can you develop the right team behind you? What's working well and what is not?
- What roles are not being fulfilled at the moment? E.g. Financial/ personal/ marketing/ editor/ promoter/ web developer/ contractors or outside skill services
- Do you need to write a checklist that is visible for your team to view?
- How can you/your team adapt quickly?
- How are you enhancing self/staff skills and professional expertise?
- How do you problem-solve specific challenges that confront your business regularly/systematically?
- How can you ensure that day-to-day work goals are directed at increasing your business's everyday effectiveness?
- Do you have a checklist of how to improve/achieve what you want to attain in the future?
- Do you have a checklist on how to come back to focus when doing boring tasks?
- Can you be transparent about what areas of the business need improving? Can you seek professional help to turn it around as quickly as possible? E.g. money/health/personal interruptions/motivation
- Do you have a checklist to conserve/carry forward what you want to hang on to?
- How do you checklist how to improve booking in performances?
- How do you document all follow up systems?
- How do you eliminate what you want to get rid of/how to steer clear of what you want to avoid?
- How many working hours with clients/on business per week will you need?
- What needs to change in communication systems? Incoming communication methods: answering emails/phone calls? Is it done as they come in or at a designated time of day?
- What can be automated in your business? E.g. bills/promotions/passive income/customer booking system
- How do you display your current first aid/business professional indemnity insurance certificates?
- How do you keep records of continuing professional education? Are you meeting the standard requirements?
- How can you arrange to provide health fund rebates? What is your procedure for health fund receipts?
- How do you establish your professional conduct? Is it congruent with your outside behaviours?
- Do you need to improve on your formal complaints procedure?
- How can you keep all staff 100% aware of business policies?
- How can all staff know the consequences of out of bounds behaviour? E.g. prescribing medication/herbs/supplements/internal examinations/massage breasts/ manipulations/ ingesting essential oils/ skin penetration including needles, piercing, tattooing
- How can you ensure the standards of work health and safety are adhered to?

Business Planning

- How can you ensure patient confidentiality? Do you need to upgrade your patient record storage? E.g. who has access to the records? Does the practitioner keep these records or does the business?
- Do you need to improve your 'in person'/telephone/internet consultations e.g. booking systems?
- How can you provide mobile service/home visits?
- How can you/team member have access to or speak another language?
- What steps need to be taken so all staff have residency or permit to work in country?
- How can you make the clinic details and location clear/easy to understand or read?
- How can individual's personal/private information be stored for easy access whilst being private?
- How can sensitive information or an opinion about an individual be handled? E.g. Racial or ethnic origin/religious beliefs/philosophical beliefs/sexual orientation or practices/health information
- How can the professional stance on personal information for the purposes of marketing and online be handled?
- How can you improve your approach to the storage & disclosure of personal information?
- How can you improve your approach to the disclosure of personal information to people overseas?
- How can you ensure that staff understands your guidelines of when they must legally inform police of 'private' information? E.g. personal harm to another/intended damage to person or property
- How can you have a system for making sure your computers/websites/plugins are updated to the latest versions to circumvent bugs and hackers?
- How can you work with debt collectors to recover income?
- How can you display refund policies?
- Can you display on your invoice reminders about paying on time?
- Do you need to review whether you have the right book keeper/accountant to support your business financially?
- Can you instantly account for how much you currently have in your business savings?
- How can you budget for your tax obligations?
- How can you budget for your monthly expenses? Do you need to borrow money for this? E.g. Marketing/travel/launderings/courses/
- Conferences/meals/electrical/wages/debts/running expenses
- How can you measure unique/new visitors to your web/facility?
- How can you measure therapy specific direct visits?
- How can you measure audience share visits from social media?
- In what way can you acknowledge customer leads?
- Do you need to review how you store old client records safely?
- Do you need to review how you store business sales/purchase records?
- How can your financial budget cater for all your business needs?
- How can you give yourself a wage from your business?
- Can your accounting system be able to do all that you need? Access statistics on income/expenses/taxes/products/services/other?
- How can your sales, administrations of order receipts/order track proficiently in the future? E.g. Automated/current/professional looking
- Have you automated as much as you can? E.g. out of office email/social media posts/reminders/paying bills/regular electronic backing up of important documents/client bookings/ticket sales. Will your automated systems actually free up your time?

- Can you have a filing system in the cloud for all your digital documents/files/photographs/brochures/client handouts/reference material?
- Can you have a physical manual filing system for all your documents/files/photographs/brochures/client handouts/reference material?
- Can you update/convert any out-dated systems seamlessly or do you have to wait for the financial year completion?
- Do you need to review your system for emails/snail mail?
- Can you manage how many days off you/your team take off for health/courses?
- What percentage of the week is working on the business/in the business?
- Do you have a system to ensure you have all your business registrations up to date? E.g. associations
- Do you need to review that you have the right business or company structure set up based on your legal and ownership structure, company size, business location, depending if it is virtual or brick-and-mortar businesses? E.g. sole trader/company/partnership/trust
- Do you need to put a business exit strategy in place? What is your legacy?
- How can you have a current written plan for your business if you/team member suffers from illness/accident/death/sudden departure? Where is that stored and who has access to it?
- How can you have all the insurances that you need?
- Professional liability insurance: covers against negligence claims due to harm that results from mistakes or failure to perform
- Property insurance: in the event of fire, storm, or theft to cover equipment/signage/inventory/furniture
- Workers' compensation insurance to cover medical treatment, disability and death benefits in the event an employee is injured or dies as a result of his work with your business
- Home-based business insurance:
- Product liability insurance: Tailored specifically to your business product to make sure it is publicly safe
- Vehicle Insurance (third-party or comprehensive) for all company vehicles to protect against liability if an accident occurs
- Business interruption insurance: If your business's physical location has a disaster or catastrophe, and your business suffers from lost income due to your staff's inability to work in the office, manufacture products or make sales calls

Mental

- What can you change so you can easily sell your products/services from your website?
- What mail-out list can you use? Is it easy to get around in? E.g. Mail chimp
- Do you know what subscriptions/plans/rentals you have, and do you use them all effectively? E.g. iCloud/Dropbox/automated social media organiser/Evernote/mobile phone plans/office equipment rentals
- How can you store all your passwords safely as a physical hard copy and on a storage app? Who else needs to know how to access them if needed?
- How will you achieve your income goals for the next 4/6/12 months?
- What passive income will/are you able to create this next 4/6/12 month period?
- How are you going to educate yourself more about financial strategies? E.g. Read books/webinars/courses/make a budget/ track money/learn about stock markets/talk to an accountant or book keeper/electronic book keeping app/consolidate superannuation/podcasts
- Do you need to review your current standard operation procedures to provide a starting point and save time? Is everyone aware of them and how they function? E.g. business correspondence: font/margins/header and footer/emails/signatures
- How can all staff know the policy procedures for bookings/cancelations and refunds?
- Do you need to review your system that handles paper and electronic invoices and receipts?
- How are you prepared ahead of time, knowing when to submit taxes?
- Is your business always ready for an audit?
- How can your costing structure be proficient?
- Can you have financial/accounting workflow tracking for daily/weekly/monthly/yearly jobs?
- Do you know how to translate your profit and loss statements?
- How can productivity be translated into dollar value? E.g. procrastination/skill level?
- How do you map current business baseline?
- How can you ensure your organisational structure is congruent with productivity and income?
- How can you track sales and guarantee delivery date?
- How can your product/service make news that people would travel from across the world to experience?
- How are you asking for help in the areas that you find difficult or time consuming?
- What procedure is in place when part of your product/service breaks? How soon before it can be corrected?
- How can you manage your team more effectively? Is your management style directive/authoritive/affiliative/participative/pace setting or coaching (see Appendix 4)

REVIEW

Yay!!! You did it!!! You have finished your planning; you have set deadlines and schedules. You have made specific goals, scheduled them into your diary and run your business for some time with your new goals.

This review section is where you now check how you went against your goals.

On your 7-10 goals you aimed for:

Did you reach your goals?

If yes, yay!!! Party time. Remember it's important to celebrate your successes.

If goals and objectives were not reached, what are you going to do about it? Was it due to finances, time, marketing, knowledge or resources?

Do you need to adjust or reschedule your goals? Goals can be changed at any time to adapt to your changing environment.

A new focus is reaffirmed for the future.

Reach for the stars, have the business you always dreamed of.

Love This Life

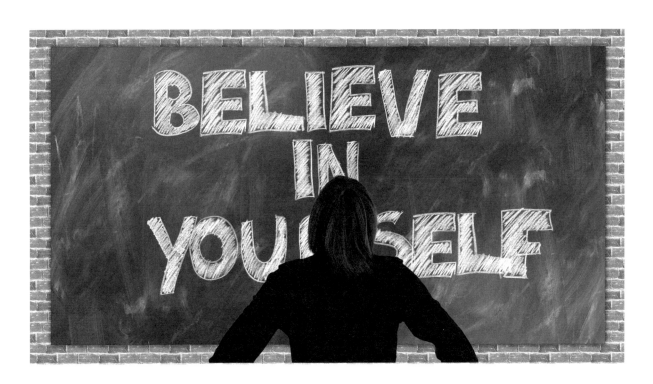

APPENDIX 1 – AVATAR ANALYSIS

Use this form to help you narrow down who you want to target

Male/Female/Both		Age Range:	
Number of Children:		Age of Children:	
Number of Pets:		Type of Pets:	
Extended family still living with them		Parents/Grown Up Children	

LEISURE & LIFESTYLE

Number of times per year they holiday	
Where do they go?	Local/ Interstate/ Family/ Overseas
How long do they Holiday?	Weekend/ Weekly/ Months
How much money do they spend on holidays?	Budget/Moderate/Extravagant

FINANCE AND LEGAL ISSUES

Housing	Renting/Own/Own More than One House/Multi Dwelling Accommodation/No Fixed Location
Schooling	Nil/Part Time/Full Time
Where do they buy?	Online/Department Store/Market/Direct
Reason to Purchase	Cheap/Convenient/Ethical/Fresh/Original/Keeping up with the Jones
Where do they spend most of their money?	Health and Beauty/Personal Possessions/ Educational/Holidays/Other People

HEALTH AND FITNESS

Level of fitness	0-10/10	Number of exercise hours per week:	0-Professional Athletic
Where do they exercise		Home/ Gym/ Indoors/ Outdoors/ Privately/ Group Training	
What % do they spend monthly on		Health/Exercise Clothing/Organic or Ethical Food	

SPIRITUALITY

Religious/Spiritual/Atheist	

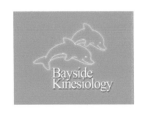

CONTACT
Bayside Kinesiology Brisbane,
Queensland AUSTRALIA

http://www.baysidekinesiology.com
ranee.zeller@baysidekinesiology.com

PH: 0419 737 396

LIFESTYLE AND HOUSING

Prefer to be	Indoors/Outdoors
Do they own items or do they have access to Things/Experiences	
Size of Housing Accommodation	Mansion/Average/Minimalist/No Fixed Location

PAID WORK

Income per week	Minimal/Average Wage/Above Standard/Fluctuates/Passive
Reason for work	Pay Bills/Family and Pet Commitments /Holidays/Health/Retirement Saving/Accumulation of Assets

NON-PAID WORK

Number of hours per week		Number of days per week of volunteer work	1-7
Reason for Community/Volunteer Work		Give Back/ Sharing Skills/ People Interaction/ Loneliness	

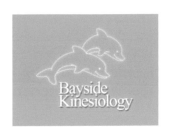

CONTACT
Bayside Kinesiology Brisbane,
Queensland AUSTRALIA

http://www.baysidekinesiology.com
ranee.zeller@baysidekinesiology.com

PH: 0419 737 396

Appendix

APPENDIX 2 – MISSION STATEMENTS

Amazon

"To be Earth's most customer-centric company, where customers can find and discover anything they might want to buy online, and endeavours to offer its customers the lowest possible prices."

Apple

"Apple is committed to bringing the best personal computing experience to students, educators, creative professionals and consumers around the world through its innovative hardware, software and Internet offerings."

Coca Cola

To Refresh the World... in body, mind, and spirit. To inspire moments of optimism and happiness...To Create Value and Make a Difference...

Disney

"We create happiness by providing the finest in entertainment for people of all ages, everywhere"

Facebook

"Facebook's mission is to give people the power to share and make the world more open and connected."

Google

'To make the world's information universally accessible and useful'

McDonald's

"To be our customers' favourite place and way to eat and drink. Our worldwide operations are aligned around a global strategy called the Plan to Win, which centre on an exceptional customer experience – People, Products, Place, Price and Promotion. We are committed to continuously improving our operations and enhancing our customers' experience"

Red Cross

"The International Committee of the Red Cross (ICRC) is an impartial, neutral and independent organization whose exclusively humanitarian mission is to protect the lives and dignity of victims of armed conflict and other situations of violence and to provide them with assistance. The ICRC also endeavours to prevent suffering by promoting and strengthening humanitarian law and universal humanitarian principles."

Starbucks

"To inspire and nurture the human spirit – one person, one cup and one neighbourhood at a time."

Twitter

"To instantly connect people everywhere to what's most important to them"

Walmart

"We save people money so they can live better."

Whole Foods Market

"Our deepest purpose as an organization is helping support the health, well-being, and healing of both people — customers, Team Members, and business organizations in general — and the planet."

APPENDIX 3 – SAMPLE CODE OF CONDUCT/ETHICS

Below is a typical example of a code of conduct from a "Natural Therapy Industry."

A code of conduct/ethics is a public statement developed for and by the health profession to:
- Clarify what constitutes unprofessional conduct
- Indicate to the community the values, which are expected of its members

Therefore, the Code of Conduct was established as the basis for ethical and professional conduct in order to meet community expectations and justify community trust in the judgement and integrity of its members.

While the Code of Conduct is not underpinned in statute, adoption and adherence to it by its members, it is a condition of all membership. A breach of the Code of Conduct may render a member liable for removal from the Register of Members.

1. Ethical Principles
- Practitioners conduct themselves ethically and professionally at all times
- Practitioners render their professional services in accordance with holistic principles for the benefit and wellbeing of patients
- Practitioners do no harm to patients
- Practitioners have a commitment to continuing professional education to maintain and improve their professional knowledge, skills and attitudes
- Practitioners respect an individual's autonomy, needs, values, culture and vulnerability in the provision of complementary medicine treatment
- Practitioners accept the rights of individuals and encourage them to make informed choices in relation to their healthcare, and support patients in their search for solutions to their health problems
- Practitioners recognise their limitations and the competence of other healthcare professionals, and when indicated, recommend that additional opinions and services be sought
- Practitioners treat all patients with respect, and do not engage in any form of exploitation for personal advantage whether financial, physical, sexual, emotional, religious or for any other reason

2. Duty of Care
- The highest level of professional and ethical care shall be given to patients
- The practitioner will exercise utmost care to avoid unconscionable behaviour
- The patient has the right to receive treatment that is provided with skill, competence, diligence and care
- In the exercise of care of the patient, the practitioner shall not misrepresent or misuse their skill, ability or qualification

3. Professional Conduct

- Practitioner members must adhere to all of the requirements of this Code of Conduct and State, Territory and Federal law within the scope of their practice
- Practitioners (who are not registered medical practitioners) who choose to adopt the title "Dr" in advertising, whether or not they hold a Doctorate or PhD, to make it clear that they do not hold a registration as a medical practitioner. In their advertising the title of "Doctor" or "Dr" will not be used, unless registered with an Australian medical registration board. In advertising they should include a reference to their health profession whenever the title is used
- Under no circumstances may a student, staff member or another practitioner use someone else's membership number or tax invoice book for purposes of issuing a health fund rebate tax invoice. The practitioner is responsible for the issue of their own tax accounting
- The practitioner shall not provide false, misleading or incorrect information regarding health fund rebates, work cover, or any other documents
- The practitioner shall not advertise under a false logo any discipline/s for which they are not accredited
- The practitioner shall not denigrate other members of the healthcare profession
- The practitioner shall be responsible for the actions of all persons under their employ, whether under contract or not
- The practitioner shall not engage in activity, whether written or verbal, that will reflect improperly on the profession
- In the conveying of scientific or empirical knowledge to a patient, the practitioner shall act responsibly, and all personal opinions shall be highlighted as such
- Students shall not engage in clinical practise other than as part of supervised training. In all other student obligations, students must identify themselves as such and not charge a fee
- In the clinical setting, the practitioner shall not be under the influence of any substance capable of impairing professional judgement
- The medicines and medical devices used by the practitioner must be in accordance with therapeutic goods law
- Telephone/Internet/online audio-visual consultations can be conducted for approved modalities
- The fee for service and medicines (where qualified) charged by the practitioner must be reasonable, avoiding any excess or exploitation.

4. Relationship Between Practitioner and Patient

- The practitioner shall not discriminate on the basis of race, age, religion, gender, ethnicity, sexual preference, political views, medical condition, socioeconomic status, culture, marital status, physical or mental disability
- The practitioner must behave with courtesy, respect, dignity and discretion towards the patient, at all times respecting the diversity of individuals and honouring the trust in the therapeutic relationship
- The practitioner should assist the patient find another healthcare professional if required
- Should a conflict of interest or bias arise, the practitioner shall declare it to the patient, whether the conflict or bias is actual or potential, financial or personal

5. Professional Boundary

- The practitioner will not enter into an intimate or sexual relationship with a patient
- The practitioner will not engage in contact or gestures of a sexual nature to a patient
- Mammary glands and genitalia of a patient will not be touched or massaged and only professional techniques applied to surrounding tissue
- Any internal examination of a patient, even with the consent of the patient, is regarded as indecent assault, which is a criminal offence
- Any approaches of a sexual nature by a patient must be declined and a note made in the patient's record

6. Personal Information and Confidentiality

- The practitioner will abide by the requirements of State, Territory and Federal privacy and patient record law
- The practitioner shall honour the information given by a patient in the therapeutic relationship
- The practitioner shall ensure that there will be no wrongful disclosure, either directly or indirectly, of a patient's personal information
- Patient records must be securely stored, archived, passed on or disposed of in accordance with State, Territory and Federal patient record law
- Appropriate measures shall be in place to ensure that patient information provided by facsimile, email, mobile telephone or other media shall be secure
- Patient records must be properly maintained with adequate information of a professional standard.
- The practitioner must act with due care and obtain consent when conveying a patient's information to another healthcare professional
- The patient has a right to be adequately informed as to their treatment plan and medicines, and access to their information as far as the law permits

7. Advertising

- Advertisements, in any form of printed or electronic media, must not:
- Be false, misleading or deceptive
- Abuse the trust or exploit the lack of knowledge of consumers
- Make claims of treatment that cannot be substantiated
- Make claims of cure
- Use the title of Doctor, unless registered with an Australian medical registration board
- Encourage excessive or inappropriate use of medicines or services

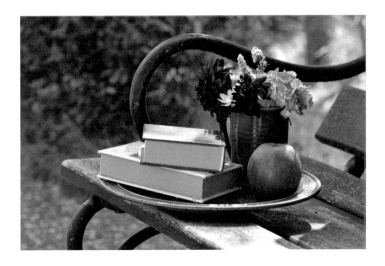

APPENDIX 4 – THE 6 MANAGEMENT STYLES

According to Hay-McBer there are six key leadership or management styles https://leadersinheels.com/career/6-management-styles-and-when-best-to-use-them-the-leaders-tool-kit/

Directive

The directive (Coercive) style has the primary objective of immediate compliance from employees:

- The "do it the way I tell you" manager
- Closely controls employees
- Motivates by threats and discipline

Effective when:

- There is a crisis
- When deviations are risky

Least effective when:

- Employees are underdeveloped – little learning happens with this style
- Employees are highly skilled – they become frustrated and resentful at the micromanaging.

Authoritative

The authoritative (Visionary) style has the primary objective of providing long-term direction and vision for employees:

- The "firm but fair" manager
- Gives employees clear direction
- Motivates by persuasion and feedback on task performance

Effective when:

- Clear directions and standards needed
- The leader is credible

Least effective when:

- Employees are underdeveloped – they need guidance on what to do
- The leader is not credible – people won't follow your vision if they don't believe in it

Affiliative

The affiliative style has the primary objective of creating harmony among employees and between manager and employees:

- The "people first, task second" manager
- Avoids conflict and emphasises good personal relationships among employees
- Motivates by trying to keep people happy

Effective when:

- Used with other styles
- Tasks routine, performance adequate
- Counselling, helping
- Managing conflict

Least effective when:

- Performance is inadequate – affiliation does not emphasise performance
- There are crisis situations needing direction

Participative

The participative (Democratic) style has the primary objective of building commitment and consensus among employees:
- The "everyone has input" manager
- Encourages employee input in decision making
- Motivates by rewarding team effort

Effective when:
- Employees working together
- Staff have experience and credibility
- Steady working environment

Least effective when:
- Employees must be coordinated
- There is a crisis – no time for meetings
- There is a lack of competency – close supervision required

Pacesetting

The pacesetting style has the primary objective of accomplishing tasks to a high standard of excellence:
- The "do it myself" manager
- Performs many tasks personally and expects employees to follow his/her example
- Motivates by setting high standards and expects self-direction from employees

Effective when:
- People are highly motivated, competent
- Little direction/coordination required
- When managing experts

Least effective when:
- When workload requires assistance from others
- When development, coaching & coordination required

Coaching

The coaching style has the primary objective of long-term professional development of employees:
- The "developmental" manager
- Helps and encourages employees to develop their strengths and improve their performance
- Motivates by providing opportunities for professional development

Effective when:
- Skill needs to be developed
- Employees are motivated and wanting development

Least effective when:
- The leader lacks expertise
- When performance discrepancy is too great – coaching managers may persist rather than exit a poor performer

APPENDIX 5 – NEGATIVE BUSINESS BELIEFS

Rich people are:

- Ambitious/Greedy/Snobs/Arrogant/Condescending/Aloof/Judgemental
- Love power
- Love seeing themselves as superior
- Love things and use people (exploit, take advantage of)
- Manipulate others to get what they want by being dominant aggressive or sly; using guile, charm, charisma, bullying or intimidation
- Are desensitised to how others may feel about the 'deal', experience or the emotional/psychological environment they are placed in
- Have no care or concern for others (narcissistic behaviour) or whom they hurt in accomplishing their agenda. As long as they get what they want
- Are corrupt. (Financial advisors, investment gurus, share portfolio spruikers)
- Are conniving schemers who want access to the resources others have worked hard for all their life
- Just walk away and start again when things fail. They ruin people i.e. mums & dads who invest their home to help fund their pension and they lose everything and are left destitute
- Get away with it because they transfer this money off shore or into family trusts. Have the mansion by the beach; the boat, the holidays and innocent hopeful, well-intentioned people are left destitute
- Focused on/obsessed with getting more, accumulate for the sake of it. Always more, they don't need it. They just want – want- want, never satisfied
- Have "Short arms – long pockets", meaning they love to receive but won't give.
- Expect others to pick up the tab, or to give to them. Can't be generous. "I can't afford a coffee. Oh, your shout – sure!"   Hoarding nature

Perceptions

- Are only interested in me if they can get something from me otherwise I'm invisible
- Do not include me in their exclusive, elitist club
- Reject me. Their attitude appears to be "I'm not good enough' because I haven't accomplished the things that are important. E.g. expensive car, right postcode, home with a view, status career, trophies or accolades. In their eyes I'm a nobody, a loser causing me to feel ashamed of who I am

They view me as:

- Not successful
- Not intelligent enough
- Not of their standard: e.g. not a trophy or bauble to hang of their arm
- I'm not a thoroughbred. Too short, too dumpy, too mediocre, too …. etc.

I don't deserve it because I:

- Am lazy, apathy, not smart or shrewd enough, not good at school/scholastics (e.g. not a doctor or lawyer)
- Can't impress people – can't think on my feet
- Don't have the gift of the gab
- Am not charming
- Always offend people – say the wrong thing
- Hate being taken advantage of – for granted
- Am stubborn
- Won't play the game
- Won't let other people play me/use me
- Reject successful businessmen before they reject me
- Don't even want to mix with the likes of them
- Don't want to have to do what it takes
- Was born under an unlucky star
- Have bad karma
- Did not have success in my path/blue print
- Married the wrong guy
- Had the wrong parents
- Inherited bad genes
- Have ADHD/dyslexia
- Am shy
- Don't want to be noticed
- Want to remain invisible
- Let positive thought (wishful thinking) do all the work
- People don't really want to know me and avoid me
- I attract the underdogs not the winners
- Give – they take – I am used

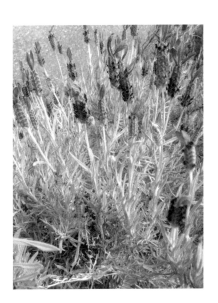

Appendix

What is the ideal…. Hopes and Dreams

- I will have money when I get my inheritance
- I don't have to compromise my integrity, value system, or comfortable behaviour to acquire money. I just receive from a source. No effort required. Instant abundance
- My spouse is driven and successful and I will reap the rewards/benefits
- I will have a big house, holidays o/s, toys, no need to work
- I am lucky
- I will achieve wealth through innovation
- I will have an idea and invent something that changes the worked e.g: post it notes or Velcro
- I have gifted genes/God/a fluke
- I will be discovered
- I will be successful through my beauty/art/athletic ability
- I will spend my life doing what I love to do
- I will produce something the rich want e.g: works of art or new technology or app
- I never put a foot wrong – lady luck is on my side
- I always buy before a boom
- I am good at coming across a fixer-upper for profit
- I will buy shares that skyrocket

APPENDIX 6 – WORK HEALTH AND SAFETY

INTRODUCTION TO HEALTH AND SAFETY IN THE WORKPLACE

[Company] t/a [Company] **(the Organisation)** will do everything reasonably practicable to ensure that workers can undertake their work in a healthy and safe manner. We all play a crucial role in achieving a workplace that is free of injury and illness. The Organisation will work towards achieving this goal by providing workers with the necessary resources.

PURPOSE OF THE HEALTH AND SAFETY MANUAL

The purpose of this Health and Safety Manual is to establish the minimum standards and guidelines that are reasonably practicable for this Organisation to manage the hazards and risks in the workplace. In addition to this manual, the Organisation utilises a Health and Safety Handbook and a number of forms to assist in managing health and safety.

These standards will provide greater consistency, certainty and clarity across the Organisation to make it easier to understand health and safety duties and responsibilities.

All workers will be given the opportunity to read this information and are encouraged to participate in following and improving health and safety in the Organisation.

HEALTH AND SAFETY POLICY STATEMENT

[Company] t/a [Company] and its officers recognise that the health and safety of all workers and visitors is of the utmost importance and vital to the success of our business. As such we aim to continuously improve health and safety in the workplace through consultation and increased health and safety awareness of management and workers.

Through the co-operative efforts of management and workers, we are committed to:
* Providing a safe environment for all workers and visitors to our workplace
* Providing and maintaining buildings, plant and equipment in safe working condition
* Supporting the on-going training and assessment of workers
* Developing, implementing and monitoring safe work practices
* Continuously improving the standards of health and safety in the workplace
* Managing risks in the workplace
* Providing information, instruction and supervision.

The focus of [Company] t/a [Company] health and safety management system is preventing hazards. We will develop a framework for health and safety management and a plan for systematic risk assessment and control of hazards, to progressively improve safe behaviours and safe systems of work across the business.

[Director/Manager]
Director

on behalf of [Company] t/a [Company]
Date: [Date]
Review date: [Date]

HEALTH AND SAFETY RESPONSIBILITIES

ORGANISATION'S RESPONSIBILITIES

The Organisation has a duty to ensure, so far as reasonably practicable, the health and safety at work of all its workers. In particular, it is responsible for:

- Providing and maintaining its workplaces in a healthy and safe condition and providing safe systems of work
- Identifying, controlling and monitoring hazards in the workplace
- Ensuring the safe use, handling, storage and transportation of plant, equipment and substances
- Providing and maintaining systems of work and a working environment that is healthy and safe
- Providing the information, training, instruction and supervision necessary to maintain a healthy and safe workplace
- Providing adequate facilities for the welfare of workers
- Monitoring the workplace and the health and safety of workers to assist in preventing injury and illness.

MANAGER/SUPERVISOR RESPONSIBILITIES

Managers/supervisors are responsible for:

- Maintaining a working environment that is safe and without risk to health
- Implementing safe systems of work by ensuring safe products and systems are used
- Maintaining the workplace, plant, machinery and substances
- Implementing the information, training, instruction and supervision for workers
- Identifying and controlling hazards in the workplace
- Ensuring all relevant health and safety laws are complied with
- Using the resources provided for health and safety
- Ensuring workplace rules, procedures and systems are reviewed and maintained
- Promoting health and safety in the workplace
- Maintaining consultative mechanisms.

WORKER RESPONSIBILITIES

Workers are responsible for:

- Ensuring they are not under the influence of alcohol, drugs or medication of any kind where doing so could adversely affect their ability to perform their duties safely or efficiently or be in breach of the workplace policies
- Taking reasonable care for the health and safety of themselves and others who may be affected by their actions or omissions in the workplace
- Co-operating with management to ensure all health and safety obligations are complied with
- Ensuring all health and safety equipment is used correctly
- Using and maintaining the required personal protective equipment (PPE)
- Reporting any incidents or injuries sustained while working and seeking appropriate first aid
- Reporting any unsafe conditions, equipment or practices to management, as soon as practicable
- Rectifying minor health and safety issues where authorised and safe to do so
- Co-operating with any health and safety initiative, inspection or investigation
- Actively participating in any return to work program.

CONSULTATION

CONSULTATION STATEMENT

- The Organisation is committed to protecting the health and safety of all its workers. Injury and illness are needless, costly and preventable.
- The Organisation will consult with workers regarding the implementation of practices and systems that will ensure the health and safety of workers. Worker involvement at all levels is essential for ensuring a healthy and safe workplace.
- The Organisation's health and safety consultation arrangements fall into the generic category of 'Agreed Arrangements'.
- The primary medium for consultation is direct dialogue between management and workers. Consultation at this level is fundamental to the successful management of health and safety risks.
- Consultation on health and safety issues must be meaningful and effective to allow each worker to contribute to decisions that may affect their health and safety at work.
- All workers will be given the opportunity to express their views and contribute in a timely manner to the resolution of health and safety issues that affect them. These views will be valued and taken into account by those making decisions.
- The consultation arrangements at the Organisation will be monitored and reviewed as the need arises to ensure they continue to be meaningful and effective.

ORGANISATION'S RESPONSIBILITIES

The Organisation will consult with workers in relation to:
- Identifying hazards and assessing risks arising from the work carried out or to be carried out
- Eliminating or minimising identified hazards and risks
- The adequacy of facilities for the welfare of workers
- Proposed changes that may affect the health and safety of workers
- Proposed changes to key health and safety policies and procedures, including those relating to consultation, dispute resolution, the monitoring of the health of workers, conditions in the workplace, and the provision of information and training for workers.

CONSULTATION PROCEDURES

Staff meetings

The Organisation recognises the involvement of workers as essential in identifying potential hazards that can be eliminated or minimised before injuries occur. To facilitate this, the Organisation will make health and safety an agenda item at regular staff meetings.

Staff/team meetings will be used to:

- Notify and remind workers of health and safety policies and procedures
- Provide a forum for workers to have their say about health and safety issues
- Maintain awareness of health and safety.

Where required, specific health and safety issues will be raised, incidents and accidents reviewed, procedures developed and communicated, and health and safety alerts discussed.

Meetings will be used to induct workers into new or amended health and safety procedures and 'sign off' their understanding of the controls provided for the specific work in which they will be involved.

Appendix

If a worker is absent from a staff meeting, the worker will be provided with any relevant information and training upon their return to work.

Team Toolbox Meetings and Communication

To assist in the identification and control of hazards, the Organisation will conduct toolbox meetings at regular intervals and on an 'as needed' basis.

Toolbox meetings will be conducted to help supervisors manage safety, to provide a forum for workers to have their say about safety issues and to help ensure safety awareness is maintained. Where required, specific safety issues will be raised, accidents reviewed, Safe Work Method Statements (**SWMS**) and/or Safe Work Procedures (**SWP**) developed and presented for evaluation and familiarisation, and safety alerts discussed.

Toolbox meetings will also be used to induct workers into and 'sign off' their understanding of the controls provided in the **SWMS/SWP**s for the specific work for which they will be involved in. All toolbox meetings will be recorded on the **Toolbox Talk form** and signed off by participants. Where corrective actions are identified, these will be followed up and signed off by the nominated person.

Noticeboards

A health and safety noticeboard will be positioned in a conspicuous place in the workplace. The noticeboard will display the following:

- The Organisation's Health and Safety Policy
- Information regarding the Organisation's **Injury Management and Return-to-Work** program, which should be reviewed and amended in line with any specific requirements of your workers compensation insurer
- Copies of the Organisation's Incident Report Form and Hazard Report Form
- The Organisation's agreed Safety Consultation Statement outlining the agreed arrangements for reporting and managing safety issues
- A list of designated first aid personnel and their contact details
- A list of emergency wardens.

In addition, minutes of the most recent staff meeting should be displayed on the noticeboard.

In addition, minutes of the most recent toolbox meeting should be displayed on the noticeboard.

RISK MANAGEMENT PROCESS

INTRODUCTION

Risk management is the key process in ensuring a safe and healthy workplace. In health and safety terms, risk management is the process of identifying situations which have the potential to cause harm to people or property, and then taking appropriate steps to prevent the hazardous situation occurring or reduce the risk of injury to workers.

The Organisation has a duty to undertake risk management activities to ensure the health and safety of its workers, contractors, visitors and others in the workplace. The Organisation will as far as is reasonably practicable, ensure that the workplace is free from hazards that could cause injury or illness.

Control of hazards takes a variety of forms depending on the nature of the hazard and must be based on the hierarchy of control options emphasising the elimination of the hazard at its source.

THE RISK MANAGEMENT PROCESS

The risk management process consists of four well-defined steps. These are as follows:

Step 1: *Identifying* - Identifying the problem, this is known as hazard identification

Step 2: *Assessing* - Determining how serious a problem it is, the likelihood of an incident/accident occurring and the consequence and potential severity, this is known as risk assessment

Step 3: *Controlling* - Deciding what needs to be done to solve the problem, this is known as risk elimination or control

Step 4: *Monitoring and Review* – This involves reviewing the actions taken to determine the effectiveness of the controls implemented.

Hazard Identification

Hazard identification aims to determine what hazards exist (or could foreseeably exist), so that control measures can be implemented to address the hazard before it causes any harm.

Hazard identification activities will include:

- Conducting workplace inspections to identify hazards
- Regular work area observations and discussions with workers
- Identifying and assessing hazards on an ongoing basis
- Assessing products and services prior to purchasing to identify potential risks
- Undertaking incident and injury investigations and reviewing past incident and accidents data
- Talking to workers performing the task to find out what they consider as safety issues
- Reviewing any information already available, for example safety data sheets, manufacturer's specifications and instructions and safe operating procedure to see what hazards have already been identified and how these are controlled
- Thinking creatively about what could happen if something went wrong.

Identified hazards will be recorded on a Hazard Report Form or **Risk Register** which will be used in conjunction with the monitoring and review of identified hazards and implemented controls.

Risk Assessment

Once a hazard has been identified, the Organisation, in consultation with workers, will conduct a Risk Assessment to determine how likely it is that someone could be harmed by the hazard and how serious the injury or illness could be. The risk assessment will be recorded on the **Risk Assessment Form**.

If a hazard is obvious and the risk of injury or illness is high, action will be taken immediately to control the risk, even if only as an interim measure. Where a control is implemented as an interim measure, a thorough risk assessment will be conducted to decide on more permanent control measures.

When assessing the risk of injury or illness the following information regarding the hazard will be reviewed where relevant:

- Any hazard information supplied with a product or substance such as safety data sheets
- Workers experience with similar hazards or from incident/injury data
- Guidance materials available from government health and safety bodies/regulators in relation to particular hazards, processes or work tasks
- Industry codes of practice
- Relevant Australian standards

Appendix

- The working environment, including the layout and condition of the premises and equipment and the materials used in the workplace
- The capability, skill, experience and age of people ordinarily undertaking the work
- The training, supervision and work procedures being used
- Any reasonably foreseeable changes in the working conditions and environment.

Once the above information has been considered, an initial risk ranking can be applied to the hazard to enable the Organisation to set priorities for control measures. The Risk Ranking Matrix is used to provide a priority list for control actions. The Initial Risk Ranking is recorded for each hazard on the **Risk Assessment Form.**

Identified risks and any control measures implemented should be recorded on a **Risk Register** which will be used to assist in the monitoring and review process.

Risk assessments undertaken for specific tasks/items will be recorded in the **Risk Assessment Record form**.

i) Hazard Elimination or Risk Control

Once the hazards in the workplace have been identified and assessed, priorities will be set determining what action is to be taken to eliminate or control the hazard. Control of risk takes a variety of forms depending on the nature of the hazard and should be based on the 'hierarchy of control' options emphasising the elimination of the hazard at its source, or if this is not reasonably practicable, then reducing the risks to the worker. The hierarchy of control measures will be applied when determining control measures for each identified hazard in the workplace.

Where a hazard is identified, the Organisation will use the below hierarchy to determine the most effective and appropriate control measure:
- Level 1 controls provide the highest level of health and safety protection and are the most reliable in preventing harm. They involve eliminating the hazard from the workplace, for example, by bringing a job to ground level to eliminate the need to work at heights
- Level 2 controls provide a medium level of health and safety protection, and as such will only be used if a Level 1 control is not reasonably practicable. Level 2 controls may involve:
- Substituting (either wholly or partly) the hazard from the workplace with something that presents a lesser risk. For example, substituting a non-toxic, organic cleaner for a toxic cleaner
- Isolating the hazard so that no worker is exposed to it. For example, removing power or energy from a malfunctioning piece of equipment, or blocking access to an area of the workplace deemed hazardous
- Implementing engineering solutions that reduce the risk of the hazard impacting the worker. For example, erecting a guard or barrier to prevent a worker from reaching into machinery whilst it is operating
- Level 3 controls provide the lowest level of health and safety protection, and as such will only be used if a Level 1 or Level 2 control is not reasonably practicable. These controls will be used in conjunction with a Level 2 control to reduce the risk to an acceptable level. This may involve:
- Implementing administrative controls to reduce the exposure of workers to the remaining risk. For example, training everyone to work safely, writing a safe work method statement, rotating the work or managing the time workers are exposed to the risk
- Providing PPE in conjunction with other Level 2 and Level 3 controls.

Agreed control measures should not introduce any new hazards or risks to the workplace. The implemented controls are recorded in the **Hazard/Risk Register** and on the **Risk Assessment Form** for individual tasks and items. Periodic review of control measures must be undertaken to determine their suitability and effectiveness.

INCIDENT AND INJURY REPORTING

INTRODUCTION

The reporting of incidents, injuries and near hits/misses is essential for the identification of hazards in the workplace. Depending on the nature of an incident or injury, there may also be a legal obligation to report this to a state regulatory body.

To ensure compliance with these obligations, incidents and injuries will be reported in accordance with the below procedures.

REPORTING REQUIREMENTS

All incidents resulting in or with the potential for injury or property damage will be reported. Investigations of incidents will be undertaken at a level consistent with the actual or potential for injury/damage, with the goal of preventing future occurrences.

ii)   Internal Reporting and Investigation Procedures

Minor injuries which require no treatment or first aid treatment only should be recorded in the **First Aid Treatment Log/Register of Injuries.**

An incident, injury, illness or near hit/miss that requires (or has the potential to require) medical treatment should be reported on the **Incident Report Form**. This should be done as soon as possible by the affected worker (or delegate) and no later than 24 hours after the event.

If full details of the incident, injury, investigation and corrective actions are not available within this timeframe, the essential details of the incident or injury as they are known should be submitted initially.

Reported incidents and injuries will be promptly investigated by appropriate management using the **Incident Investigation Form**. The investigation will identify the causes of the incident and assess any hazards that need to be controlled. Management will discuss the incident with relevant workers and decide on suitable risk controls to be implemented using the risk management process.

The investigation and corrective actions are to be summarised in the **Incident Report Form**.

External Reporting Requirements

The Organisation will notify the relevant state health and safety regulator immediately by phone of any dangerous or notifiable incident and will secure and not interfere with the incident site. Where a required notice in writing shall be provided within 48 hours of the event.

A dangerous or notifiable incident is:
*   An incident involving the death of a worker
*   An incident involving a serious injury or illness of a worker
*   An incident otherwise considered a dangerous incident.

A *serious injury or illness* of a worker means an injury or illness requiring the worker to have:

- Immediate treatment as an in-patient in a hospital
- Immediate treatment for
  - The amputation of any part of his or her body
  - A serious head injury
  - A serious eye injury
  - A serious burn
  - The separation of skin from an underlying tissue (such as de-gloving or scalping)
  - A spinal injury
  - The loss of a bodily function
  - Serious lacerations
  - Medical treatment within 48 hours of exposure to a substance.

A *dangerous incident* means an incident in relation to a workplace that exposes a worker or any other person to a serious risk to health and safety emanating from an immediate or imminent exposure to:

- An uncontrolled escape, spillage or leakage of a substance
- An uncontrolled implosion, explosion or fire
- An uncontrolled escape of gas or steam
- An uncontrolled escape of a pressurised substance
- Electric shock
- The fall or release from a height of any plant, substance or thing
- The collapse, overturning, failure or malfunction of, or damage to, any plant that is required to be authorised for use in accordance with applicable health and safety regulations
- The collapse or partial collapse of a structure
- The collapse or failure of an excavation or of any shoring supporting an excavation
- The inrush of water, mud or gas in workings, in an underground excavation or tunnel
- The interruption of the main system of ventilation in an underground excavation or tunnel.

In addition, the Organisation will notify its workers compensation insurer within 48 hours of any injury or illness that has the potential to result in a worker's compensation claim.

INCIDENT NOTIFICATION

One of the most important initial actions to any accident or incident is to notify those who have input, support and resources which may be required to ensure the injured worker is cared for, legislative obligations are met, and effective investigation and control measures established.

As little time as possible will be lost between the time of the accident or incident and the beginning of the response.

For significant injuries, fatalities and incidents notifiable to the authorities, management will arrange, without delay, to contact and advise the following as applicable:

- Directors/other management as soon as possible following the event and not more than 24 hours after the event
- Return to work coordinator and workers compensation claims officer
- Workers compensation insurer
- The police, where there has been a fatality

- Trauma debriefing service
- Group insurance manager (if a contractor or member of the public is injured or private property damage is sustained)
- Next of kin (either the workers manager or supervisor should communicate this information).

INJURY MANAGEMENT AND RETURN-TO-WORK

INTRODUCTION

The Organisation is committed to the return to work of workers suffering a workplace related injury or illness.

As part of this commitment, it will:

- Prevent workplace injury and illness by providing a safe and healthy working environment
- Participate in the development of an injury management plan where required and ensure that injury management commences as soon as possible after a worker is injured
- Support injured workers and ensure that early return to work is a normal expectation
- Provide suitable duties for injured workers as soon as possible
- Ensure that injured workers (and anyone representing them) are aware of their rights and responsibilities and the responsibility to provide accurate information about the injury and its cause
- Consult with workers and, where applicable, unions to ensure that the return-to-work program operates as smoothly as possible
- Maintain the confidentiality of records relating to injured workers
- Not dismiss a worker as a result of a work related injury within six months of becoming unfit for employment.

PROCEDURES

To support the above, the Organisation has established the below procedures:

1. Notification of Injuries

- All injuries must be notified to management as soon as practicable.
- All minor injuries will be recorded on the **First Aid Treatment Log/Register of Injuries**.
- All injuries requiring medical treatment must be notified to management as soon as practicable using the **Incident Report Form**.
- The Organisation's workers compensation insurers will be notified of any injuries that may require compensation within 48 hours.

2. Recovery

- All injured workers will receive appropriate first aid or medical treatment as soon as possible.
- Injured workers will be permitted to nominate a treating doctor who will be responsible for the medical management of the injury and assist in planning return to work.

3. Return to Work

- A suitable person will be arranged to explain the return to work process to injured workers.
- The injured worker will be offered the assistance of an accredited rehabilitation provider if it becomes evident that they are not likely to resume their pre-injury duties, or cannot do so without changes to the workplace or work practices.

4. Suitable Duties

- An individual return to work plan will be developed when injured workers are, according to medical advice, capable of returning to work.
- Injured workers will be provided with suitable duties that are consistent with medical advice and are meaningful, productive and appropriate to the worker's physical and psychological condition.
- Depending on the individual circumstances of injured workers, suitable duties may be at the same workplace or a different workplace, the same job with modified duties or a different job and may involve modified hours of work.

5. Non-Work Related Injury

- Where the company can accommodate a worker with a non-work related injury, it will make every endeavour to do so. A return to work plan will be developed, in consultation with the worker and his/her treating practitioner, when modified duties can be provided.

6. Dispute Resolution

- If disagreements about the return to work program or suitable duties arise, the Organisation will work with injured workers and their representatives to try to resolve the issue.
- If all parties are unable to resolve the dispute, the Organisation will seek to involve the workers compensation insurer, an accredited rehabilitation provider, the treating doctor or an injury management consultant.

7. Contacts

- The Organisation's workplace contact for return-to-work is:

Name:	Organisation:	Contact details:
[Director/Manager]	[Company]	[Phone Number]

EMERGENCY PROCEDURES

INTRODUCTION

- Building and premises emergencies may arise at any time. They can develop from a number of causes including fire, chemical spills, gas leaks, bomb threats, structural faults and civil disturbance. Any of these may threaten the safety of workers.
- The Organisation is committed to establishing and maintaining procedures to control emergency situations that could adversely affect workers.

EMERGENCY PLANS

The Organisation will ensure the workplace has procedures in place to address emergency situations.

Where necessary, emergency personnel will be nominated, trained and ready to act in an emergency situation. Training of such personnel may include attendance at emergency procedure training conducted by the building owner.

Where an emergency situation does arise, the emergency personnel will be responsible for taking control of the situation and ensuring all workers are evacuated from the workplace in accordance with the workplace emergency procedures.

Emergency evacuation exercises will be conducted annually to test emergency procedures. All workers will be required to participate in the emergency evacuation exercises. The exercises will be observed and the outcomes reviewed to determine the effectiveness of the procedures in place.

The emergency procedures will be communicated to all workers and visitors as part of the induction process.

The emergency procedure, or a summary of, should be readily accessible by workers or displayed in a prominent location within the workplace.

1. Medical Emergencies

In the event a medical emergency arises and someone requires emergency medical attention, the following procedure will be adopted:

- The situation will be assessed to ensure personnel safety
- Help will be summoned from others in the immediate vicinity, or a nominated first aid officer. The affected worker will not be left unless it is unavoidable
- The alarm will be raised and emergency services contacted. Clear instructions will be provided to emergency services on:
- The location of the worker and directions to the workplace
- The details of casualty (type of injury, age and condition of worker)
- The time of injury or illness.

2. Fire

In the event a worker discovers a fire, the following procedure will be adopted:

- The worker should assess the situation and the safety of anyone in the immediate vicinity
- The worker should immediately call for help or operate the nearest fire alarm and have someone advise the nominated emergency co-ordinator or fire warden
- Where it is safe to do so, the worker should attempt to put out the fire with a nearby fire extinguisher, aiming the extinguisher at the base of the flame
- If it is not safe to do so, the fire increases in size, or the extinguisher runs out, the worker should evacuate to the nearest evacuation assembly point.

In the event a fire alarm is sounded, the following procedure will be adopted:

- Management staff will contact emergency services
- all workers should leave the building immediately via the nearest emergency exit to the nearest evacuation assembly point
- any missing worker will be reported to a fire warden or emergency services.
- Fire exits will be kept clear from obstruction at all times. Fire extinguishers will be located in conspicuous, readily accessible locations in the workplace. A clearance of 1000mm must be maintained around each fire extinguisher. Signage that complies with AS 2444-2001 Portable fire extinguishers and fire blankets will be displayed. All workers must know their evacuation route and assembly point in case of a fire.
- At all times workers should remain calm. Workers should not run, panic or take belongings with them when evacuating. The building will not be re-entered until it has been cleared as safe to do so by the emergency co-ordinator/fire warden or emergency services.

INCIDENT REPORT

Where the workplace is affected by an emergency, the Organisation will complete an **Incident Report Form** as soon as reasonably practicable to identify the causes of the emergency, any control measures that can be implemented to prevent re-occurrence and improvements to the above emergency procedures.

FIRST AID

INTRODUCTION

First aid is the emergency care of sick or injured persons.

The Organisation is committed to providing a first aid service which satisfies its obligations under applicable health and safety legislation.

FIRST AID KITS

When considering how to provide first aid, the Organisation will consider all relevant matters including:
- The nature of the work being carried out in the workplace
- The nature of the hazards in the workplace
- The size, location and nature of the workplace
- The number and composition of workers in the workplace

First aid kits provided in the workplace will:
- Be constructed of hardy material, and if appropriate, be capable of being locked (the key being easily accessible in cases of emergency)
- Be clearly and legibly marked on the outside with the words first aid and a safety information sign complying with AS/NZS 1319
- Contain nothing except first aid equipment and resources in appropriate quantities
- Be audited on a regular basis and contents replenished as required
- Be kept clean.

The first aid kit will have attached to the inside of the lid:
- An inventory of the first aid equipment and resources which the kit is required to contain
- A notebook and pen for the purposes of recording information regarding treatment and usage
- Cardio pulmonary resuscitation (CPR) flow chart
- A **first aid treatment log/register of injuries** form, or instructions on where to obtain the form.

The Organisation will nominate a person/s, who will be responsible for monitoring and maintaining the first aid kit. The nominated person will:
- Undertake regular checks to ensure the kit contains a complete set of the required items
- Ensure any items used are replaced as soon as practicable after use
- Ensure that the contents are in good working order, have not deteriorated, are within their expiry date and sterile products are sealed and have not been tampered with
- Maintain a record of first aid kit inspection details indicating the date of inspection and the person who undertook the inspection.

FIRST AID PERSONNEL

A first aid officer will be appointed to be in charge of the first aid kit and will be readily available to render first aid when necessary.

A notice will be displayed in a prominent position near the first aid kit clearly showing:
- The name and telephone number (if applicable) of the appointed first aid officer/s
- The place where each first aid officer is normally located in the workplace.

In addition, first aid personnel will also be highlighted on the internal office extensions list.

The Organisation will designate at least one first aider for every 50 workers engaged in the workplace.

ADDITIONAL FIRST AID PERSONNEL

The Organisation will consider the following factors in determining whether additional first aid officers are required:
- The maximum number of workers in the workplace at any one time
- The nature of the work being carried out in the workplace, in particular whether workers are at a risk of being exposed to hazards that could require immediate first aid treatment
- The location and proximity of the workplace to emergency services
- The way in which work is arranged and the access each worker has to a first aider
- Any other factors that indicate that additional first aiders may be needed (for example, engaging workers on shift work, seasonal work, number of other persons in the workplace and industry specific hazards).
- Register of injuries and treatment

The Organisation will provide and maintain a workplace **First Aid Treatment Log/Register of Injuries**. Management will ensure the details of any workplace injury or illness are recorded on this register.

The register of injuries will:
- Be kept in a readily accessible area of the workplace
- Be made available for inspection when requested by an authorised inspector
- Be kept for at least five years after the date of the last entry made in it.

INCIDENT RESPONSE

The Organisation will take all steps necessary to provide emergency rescue and medical help to workers suffering a workplace related injury or illness.

Where an injury or illness requires immediate urgent attention, an ambulance will be called. When calling an ambulance, clear concise information will be relayed identifying the workers location and severity of the injury or illness.

Where the injury or illness requires the worker to leave the workplace for medical treatment, management will accompany the affected worker to provide all appropriate assistance. Where management are unavailable, another worker should accompany the affected worker, especially if there are concerns about the workers ability to travel.

Management will take any actions that will prevent or minimise the risk of further accidents, injury or property damage. For example, the accident site or equipment involved will be secured rendering it safe.

Appendix

HEALTH AND SAFETY TRAINING

INTRODUCTION

The Organisation will provide the necessary health and safety training to ensure that work can be performed in a healthy and safe manner in the workplace.

Training will focus on the hazards and risks associated with the work, along with the control measures required to ensure the health and safety of the workers.

The Organisation will ensure that no worker will commence work where they may be exposed to a hazard/s without having received the appropriate level of induction and/or training and instruction to complete the tasks safely.

AIMS OF HEALTH AND SAFETY TRAINING

The Organisation's commitment to health and safety training is communicated through the **Health and Safety Policy**.

Health and safety training is conducted to ensure that:
- Appropriate health and safety information, instruction, training and supervision is provided to all workers
- Health and safety competencies for all workers are identified and reviewed and the appropriate training provided
- Health and safety competencies of contractors, labour hire workers, volunteers and visitors are assessed prior to engagement
- Workers receive training in the health and safety requirements appropriate to their position and tasks (including re-training where necessary).

Records of training conducted will be retained by the Organisation.

HEALTH AND SAFETY TRAINING PROVIDED

The Organisation will provide the following:
- Health and safety inductions for all workers
- First aid training for nominated first aid officers
- Emergency evacuation training for nominated fire wardens if appointed
- Training on health and safety obligations for officers
- Risk management training for workers
- Skill training for plant and equipment.

A record of training will be kept using the **Skills Matrix** form, detailing when a worker was trained, and if required, when the skill expires and retraining is required. For example, CPR refresher training is required every year and first aid training is required every three years.

INSPECTION AND TESTING

INTRODUCTION

A requirement of health and safety legislation is to inspect and/or test particular equipment and processes.

The Organisation will conduct inspections and testing in accordance with health and safety legislation as part of the ongoing management of hazards in the workplace.

A risk assessment will determine the frequency of the inspections if no prerequisite time frame exists.

REQUIREMENTS FOR INSPECTION AND TESTING

This Organisation will inspect and/or test the following:
- The workplace – site inspection – every six months
- Portable electrical appliances – in accordance with the outcome of the risk assessment
- Emergency procedures – at least once a year
- Plant and equipment – before every use and as per the manufacturer's recommendations.

Records of the inspection/ testing activities will be maintained on either an internal register, record/report supplied by the tester or in item specific records such as a log book or checklist

Any item failing an inspection/test will be tagged out of service and isolated from use until it has been repaired and deemed safe for use.

Items that cannot be repaired will be disposed of in an appropriate manner.

REVIEW OF INSPECTION AND TESTING INTERVALS

Inspection and testing intervals will be reviewed as follows:
- At least annually
- After an incident or accident where a failure is attributed to inadequate inspection and testing
- When manufacturer or legislative requirements change
- In response to safety alerts.

INSPECTION AND TESTING OF REGISTERED PLANT

The Organisation will ensure that the regulatory requirements for the inspection and testing of registered plant and equipment complies with the requirements of the Regulator.

DRUGS AND ALCOHOL

INTRODUCTION

The misuse of drugs or alcohol by workers can affect their health or safety, as well as that of others (including other workers and members of the general public). Drug and alcohol misuse can also have an adverse effect on work performance, behaviour or attendance at the workplace.

The Organisation is committed to ensuring the health, safety and welfare of all workers and to preventing and reducing harm associated with being impaired by drugs or alcohol at work.

The Organisation may require screening for alcohol and drugs. This may include pre-employment testing or onsite testing prior to commencing work or at random intervals. Testing may be conducted based on reasonable suspicion or following an incident or accident. The Organisation reserves the right to carry out random testing across all levels of workers. Testing may include urine and/or swab testing.

ORGANISATION'S RESPONSIBILITIES

Management will ensure these guidelines are enforced on a day to day basis. Where a Manager suspects or is informed that a worker may be unfit to perform their duties due to drug or alcohol misuse, it is management's responsibility to assess the risk and take appropriate action. This may include:

- Directing any worker away from the work area and/or to a medical practitioner nominated by the employer where it is reasonably suspected that they are under the influence of drugs or alcohol
- Arrange for on-site testing for workers accused of being under the influence of drugs and alcohol
- Arrange for transport home for any worker under the influence of drugs or alcohol
- Counsel workers who are found to be in breach of these guidelines
- Authorise appropriate assistance for a worker whose performance is affected by drugs and/or alcohol.

Where the worker is deemed to be unfit for work due to the misuse of drugs or alcohol, he or she will usually be required to take leave without pay. In some instances, workers may be allowed to take accrued personal leave instead of leave without pay. In addition, disciplinary action may be taken against the affected worker.

MANAGER/SUPERVISOR RESPONSIBILITIES

Managers/supervisors are responsible for assessing the risks associated with workers who are under the influence of drugs or alcohol in the workplace and taking appropriate action to ensure these risks are managed. This will include:

- Directing any worker reasonably suspected of being under the influence of drugs or alcohol away from the work area and/or to a medical practitioner nominated by the Organisation for the purpose of undertaking a drug and alcohol test
- Where necessary, arranging for on-site testing of any worker accused of being under the influence of drugs or alcohol
- Arranging transport home for any worker accused of being under the influence of drugs or alcohol
- Counselling workers who are found to be in breach of these guidelines

- Authorising appropriate assistance for a worker whose performance is affected by drugs or alcohol
- Initiating the appropriate disciplinary processes where any breach of this policy is identified
- Ensuring day to day compliance with this policy and any other necessary requirements to ensure health and safety in the workplace.

WORKER RESPONSIBILITIES

Workers are responsible for:
- Ensuring they are fit for duty at all times while working
- Ensuring they are not under the influence of alcohol, drugs or medication of any kind where doing so could adversely affect their ability to perform their duties safely or efficiently
- Complying with statutory limits for blood alcohol and drug content while driving any motor vehicle, or operating any machinery, in or in connection with the performance of their duties
- Questioning their doctor or pharmacist as to the potential effects or side effects when using any prescription or over-the-counter medication, and whether they are still able to perform their job safely (including driving, where applicable)
- Notifying management when using any prescription or over-the-counter medication that may impair their ability to safely and effectively perform their job
- Ensuring they do not use, possess or distribute any alcohol, drugs or medication of any kind while at work, nor use the organisation's resources to do so at any time
- Notifying management if they suspect another worker or visitor to be adversely affected by alcohol, drugs or medication of any kind
- Complying with any reasonable request by management, or an authorised tester, to undergo testing and participate in rehabilitation programs in accordance with the organisation's policy.

In addition, when working on client sites or at any other place of work, workers must comply with any site specific drug and alcohol policies.

If a worker in this situation has any doubt about how to comply with both policies, or if the policies are inconsistent, the worker should contact management for clarification as soon as possible. In the interim, the worker should refrain from any conduct which is likely to breach either of the policies.

HEALTH AND SAFETY ISSUES RESOLUTION

INTRODUCTION

Issues may arise anywhere within the Organisation in relation to health and safety matters. Often these can be resolved at the source or where the original issue is raised. However, where an issue cannot be resolved to the satisfaction of any party following consultation and discussion on the matter, an issues resolution process will ensure that the matter is resolved in a fair and equitable manner.

When a health and safety issue arise, the parties must make reasonable efforts to achieve a timely, final and effective resolution of the issue.

Any party to the issue may inform the other party of the issue as it may relate to:
- Work carried out at the workplace
- The conduct of the organisation.

When informing any other party of an issue, there must be a defined issue to resolve and the nature and scope of the issue must be identified. All parties involved in the issue must make reasonable efforts to come to an effective, timely and final solution of the matter.

ORGANISATION'S RESPONSIBILITIES

The Organisation will consult with workers to ensure that there is genuine agreement on the Issues Resolution Procedure and will ensure that:
- All workers have sufficient knowledge and understanding of the issues resolution procedures
- All issues raised are addressed in a timely and effective manner.

Where issues are raised by other parties within the Organisation that have not been resolved at the local level, the Organisation will agree to meet or communicate with all parties to the issue in a genuine attempt to resolve the issue, taking into account:
- The overall risk to workers or other parties to the issue
- The number and location of workers and other parties affected by the issue
- The measures or controls required to resolve the risk
- The person responsible for implementing the resolution measures or controls.

The Organisation will ensure that their representative to any consultation and communication designed to resolve an issue is sufficiently competent to act on its behalf, has sufficient knowledge and understanding of the issues resolution process and has the appropriate level of seniority in the decision making process.

SUPERVISOR'S RESPONSIBILITIES

When presented with a health and safety issue, the supervisor will ensure that the individual reporting the issue has completed a **Hazard Report Form** or an **Incident Report Form**. Where an issue cannot be resolved at the localised level and/or the supervisor is unable to resolve the issue through effective consultation with the worker/s affected, the matter will be escalated to the next level of management.

WORKER'S RESPONSIBILITIES

Workers are encouraged to resolve minor health and safety issues at the source of the issue, where they are authorised and it is safe to do so.

Where the issue cannot be resolved at the initial level, the issue should be raised with the supervisor of the area concerned. Every endeavour should be made to resolve health and safety matters at departmental level before referring them to the next level within the Organisation.

Where an issue raised by workers has been considered by all levels within the Organisation and cannot be effectively resolved following genuine consultation and communication, a worker or their representative may refer the health and safety issue to their industrial union, representative association or State or Territory health and safety regulator for assistance with resolution.

ISSUES RESOLUTION OUTCOMES

Where an issue is resolved, all identified health and safety issues and their subsequent resolution will be recorded to allow the Organisation to identify potential future risks and endeavour to prevent a recurrence.

Where the issue is resolved and any party to the issue requests, details of the issue and the resolution will be set out in a written agreement.

Where a written agreement is prepared:
- All parties to the issue must be satisfied that it accurately reflects the resolution
- The agreement will be provided to all people involved with the issue and/or their representative if requested.

Where an issue remains unresolved following all reasonable efforts being made to resolve it, any party to the issue can ask the regulator to appoint an inspector to assist at the workplace. Such a request can be made regardless of whether or not there is agreement about what is deemed to be reasonable efforts to resolve the issue.

HAZARDOUS MANUAL HANDLING

INTRODUCTION

Hazardous manual handling describes any work requiring a person to lift, lower, push, pull, hold, carry, move or restrain any animate or inanimate object and involves one or more of the following:
- High or sudden force
- Awkward posture
- Exposure to vibration

Some manual handling and ergonomic activities are hazardous and may cause musculoskeletal disorders. Manual handling injuries are the most common type of workplace injuries across Australia.

The Organisation and particularly the managers and supervisors have a duty to ensure that effective procedures are implemented to identify, assess and control manual handling hazards. Hazardous manual handling tasks in the workplace will be addressed via a risk management approach.

The risk management process is to be carried out in consultation with the workers who are required to perform manual handling. Representatives of workers, such as health and safety committee members or representatives, will also be consulted as required or requested.

IDENTIFYING MANUAL HANDLING HAZARDS

Manual handling hazards can be identified by:
- Observing how workers perform the work
- Reviewing injury and incident records
- Consulting with the workers performing the manual handling.

ASSESSING MANUAL HANDLING RISKS

As part of the hazard management approach, the Organisation has an obligation to ensure that any manual handling that poses a risk of injury to workers are assessed to determine the seriousness of these hazards. To assist in accurately assessing manual handling risks a checklist has been developed and needs to be completed for each identified activity. This checklist is on the **Hazardous Manual Handling Risk Assessment Form**.

In assessing risks arising from manual handling, the following factors should be taken into account:
* The positions, posture, actions and movements adopted by workers in performing manual handling
* The layout of the workplace and workstation
* The duration and frequency of tasks performed by workers
* The location of loads and distances moved manually
* The weights and forces of loads that are manually handled
* The characteristics of loads and equipment available to assist in manual handling tasks
* The skills and experience of workers who are performing manual handling tasks, along with any special needs or requirements they may have
* Any clothing (including protective clothing) that is available or worn whilst performing manual handling
* Any other factors considered relevant to the workers.

This risk assessment process is to be carried out in consultation with the workers who are required to perform manual handling. Representatives of workers, such as health and safety committee members or representatives, will also be consulted.

In assessing manual handling risks in the workplace, the **Hazardous Manual Handling Risk Assessment** will be used.

In assessing risks arising from manual handling, the following factors should be taken into account:
* The positions, posture, actions and movements adopted by workers in performing manual handling
* The layout of the workplace
* The duration and frequency of tasks performed by workers
* The location of loads and distances moved manually
* The weights and forces of loads that are manually handled
* The characteristics of loads and equipment available to assist in manual handling tasks
* The skills and experience of workers who are performing manual handling tasks, along with any special needs or requirements they may have
* Any clothing (including protective clothing) that is available or worn whilst performing manual handling
* Any other factors considered relevant to the workers.

CONTROLLING MANUAL HANDLING RISKS

The Organisation will ensure, as far as reasonably practicable, that the risks associated with manual handling in the workplace are controlled. The process of controlling manual handling risks will be determined in consultation with the workers who are required to carry out the manual handling.

In the event that manual handling has been assessed as a risk, the Organisation will redesign the manual handling to eliminate or control the risk factors and ensure that workers involved in manual handling receive appropriate training, including training in safe manual handling techniques.

Where redesign of the manual handling is not possible, the Organisation will:
- Provide mechanical aids, personal protective equipment and/or arrange for team lifting in order to reduce the risk
- Ensure that workers receive appropriate training in safe methods of manual handling appropriate for the work identified, and in the correct use of mechanical aids, protective equipment and group lifting procedures.

HAZARDOUS CHEMICALS

INTRODUCTION

Hazardous chemicals are chemicals that have the potential to harm the health and safety of any person in the workplace. This procedure will help to ensure that all relevant workers are informed about hazardous chemicals and exposures to prevent disease and injury to the workers involved in using any hazardous chemical.

SAFETY DATA SHEETS AND REGISTERS

The Organisation will maintain a current Safety Data Sheet (**SDS**) issued within the last five years for all chemicals to be used.

Before a chemical is used for a work activity, the Organisation will review the SDS to determine if the chemical is classified as hazardous.

All workers involved in the use of chemicals classified as hazardous will be provided with information and training to allow safe completion of the required task.

No chemicals will be brought to the workplace without a current SDS. Copies of the SDS will be kept in the area where the chemical is used.

Management will maintain the **Register of Hazardous Chemicals** for all chemicals used by the Organisation and provide notification to the regulator of any manifest quantities if required.

i) Safety Data Sheets and the GHS

Since 2012 Australia has transitioned to the Globally Harmonized System of Classification and Labelling of Chemicals (GHS), an international system used to classify and communicate chemical hazards.

The GHS is a system used to classify and communicate chemical hazards using internationally consistent terms and information on chemical labels and Safety Data Sheets.

Manufacturers, importers and suppliers. Health and safety laws impose a duty on manufacturers and importers of chemicals supplied to a workplace to determine if a chemical is hazardous and to correctly classify the chemical according to the GHS. Manufacturers and importers are also responsible for ensuring that correct labels and SDS are prepared for hazardous chemicals.

Suppliers may continue to supply other workplaces with stock they have on hand after 1 January 2017 providing it was manufactured or imported prior to this date and correctly labelled at that time. From 1 January 2017 suppliers should only accept stock with GHS compliant labels. Suppliers will also need to have GHS compliant SDS available from this date.

IDENTIFYING HAZARDOUS CHEMICAL RISKS

The manufacturers' SDS and labels of all chemicals will be checked prior to use to determine whether the chemical is either hazardous or dangerous, or both.

Likewise, the risks associated with storing hazardous chemicals will be considered.

ASSESSING HAZARDOUS CHEMICAL RISKS

As part of the risk management approach, the Organisation has an obligation to ensure that any chemicals that pose a risk of injury to workers are assessed to determine the seriousness of these hazards.

In assessing risks arising from chemicals, the following factors will be taken into account:
*   The nature of the chemical
*   The label and/or a current SDS for the chemical
*   The uses of the chemical
*   The storage of the chemical
*   The potential for exposure to the chemical, including through direct skin contact, inhalation

CONTROLLING HAZARDOUS CHEMICAL RISKS

The Organisation will ensure, as far as reasonably practicable, that the risks associated with hazardous chemicals are controlled. The process of controlling hazardous chemical risks will be determined in consultation with workers.

In the event that chemicals have been assessed as a risk, the Organisation will:
*   Eliminate the chemical or task if it is not essential
*   Substitute the hazardous chemical with something less hazardous
*   Isolate exposure by using barriers or distance
*   Use engineering controls, such as local exhaust ventilation or automation of the process
*   Minimise the volumes of hazardous chemicals used
*   Establish safe work practices, such as restricting access to the area, keeping the area free of clutter, replacing lids on containers, safe storage and disposal of chemicals, being prepared for spills
*   Provide spill containment systems such as spill kits or bunding appropriate to the type of chemical on site
*   Ensure that the prescribed signage is in place to inform workers, visitors and emergency personnel of the type of hazard
*   Provide instruction and supervision appropriate to the level of expertise of the worker involved
*   Provide PPE such as gloves and safety glasses as a secondary measure to supplement the other controls outlined above.

STORAGE OF HAZARDOUS CHEMICALS

The Organisation will determine safe storage requirements for hazardous chemicals in conjunction with the SDS and the risk assessment.

In storing hazardous chemicals, the Organisation will ensure that:

- Incompatible hazardous chemicals are stored at the appropriate separation distances
- Placards and signage are located on the outside of storage areas and site perimeters as required by the relevant health and safety laws and/or Australian standards
- Appropriate fire protection and other emergency equipment are provided (for example, first aid equipment, emergency eye wash and safety showers)
- Adequate lighting and ventilation and temperature control is provided in areas where hazardous chemicals are stored and/or decanted
- Hazardous chemicals are not used or stored in proximity to any water or where they can potentially be released to water, such as via stormwater drains
- All containers of hazardous chemicals are in good condition with no damage/corrosion or leaking contents wherever possible, hazardous chemicals will be stored in their original containers, labelled as supplied. When transferring chemicals or keeping them in other containers, these new containers must be compatible, suitable for the purpose and labelled. Containers, lids, caps and seals will be checked regularly for deterioration and containers replaced when necessary. Food and drink containers will not be used to store hazardous chemicals under any circumstances
- Storage requirements for the specific hazardous chemicals will be detailed in the risk assessment.

Some hazardous chemicals may also fall into the classification of dangerous goods and may be subject to requirements under the Australian Code for the Transport of Dangerous goods by Road and Rail.

The Organisation will ensure it is aware of any specific requirements of the Environmental Protection Authority relevant to any hazardous chemicals held on site or used in the conduct of its business.

DANGEROUS GOODS & COMBUSTIBLE LIQUIDS STORAGE COMPATIBILITY CHART

LABELLING OF HAZARDOUS CHEMICALS

Since 2012 Australia has transitioned to the Globally Harmonized System of Classification and Labelling of Chemicals (GHS), an international system used to classify and communicate chemical hazards.

The GHS is a system used to classify and communicate chemical hazards using internationally consistent terms and information on chemical labels and Safety Data Sheets. The GHS provides criteria for the classification of physical hazards (e.g. flammable liquids) health hazards (e.g. carcinogens) environmental hazards (e.g. aquatic toxicity).

The GHS updates the way in which information about chemical hazards is communicated to ensure safe storage, handling and disposal. The GHS uses pictograms, signal words, and hazard and precautionary statements to communicate this information.

It should be noted that Western Australia and the Australian Capital Territory have not yet mandated use of the GHS but do require chemical hazards to be communicated.

i) Pictograms

There are nine hazard pictograms in the GHS which represent the physical, health and environmental hazards.

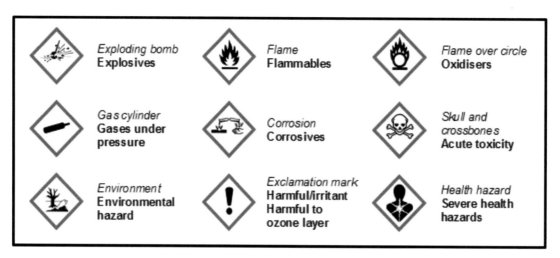

ii) Signal Words

The GHS uses 'Danger' and 'Warning' as signal words to indicate the relative level of severity of a hazard. 'Danger' is used for the more severe or a significant hazard, while 'Warning' is used for the less severe hazards.

iii) Hazard and Precautionary Statements

Hazard statements are assigned to a class and category that describes the nature of the hazards of a chemical, including, where appropriate, the degree of hazard. For example, the hazard statement 'Toxic if swallowed' is the hazard statement for Acute toxicity category 3 (Oral).

Precautionary statements describe the recommended measures that should be taken to minimise or prevent adverse effects resulting from exposure, or improper storage or handling of a hazardous chemical.

Hazard and precautionary statements replace the 'risk' and 'safety' phrases required under previous laws.

iv)   Responsibilities under the GHS

Manufacturers, importers and suppliers. Health and safety laws impose a duty on manufacturers and importers of chemicals supplied to a workplace to determine if a chemical is hazardous and to correctly classify the chemical according to the GHS. Manufacturers and importers are also responsible for ensuring that correct labels and SDS are prepared for hazardous chemicals.

Suppliers may continue to supply other workplaces with stock they have on hand after 1 January 2017 providing it was manufactured or imported prior to this date and correctly labelled at that time. From 1 January 2017 suppliers should only accept stock with GHS compliant labels. Suppliers will also need to have GHS compliant SDS available from this date.

End users of hazardous chemicals. Users of hazardous chemicals are not required to relabel or dispose of existing stock. Hazardous chemicals manufactured or imported after 1 January 2017 must only be received if they are labelled according to the requirements of the applicable health and safety regulations.

x)   Decanting and Labelling

The Organisation will ensure that any hazardous chemical decanted at the workplace is decanted into a container which is correctly labelled. The following will be displayed on the label as a minimum:
*   the product identifier
*   a hazard pictogram or hazard statement consistent with the correct classification of the hazardous chemical.

In addition to the information listed above, the Organisation will aim to provide as much information on the label as possible, pertaining to hazards and safe use of the hazardous chemical.

CONTRACTOR MANAGEMENT

INTRODUCTION

Contract workers that are engaged directly by the Organisation in core business functions and under the direct control of the Organisation are owed all the same duties and responsibilities for safety as for any other worker.

When the Organisation engages contractors in a 'contract for service' (workers are employed by another Organisation), it is important to determine the health and safety responsibilities of both parties.

The selection process for a contractor will determine whether the contractor (or sub-contractor) is able to meet the Organisation's safety expectations and ensure the well-being of workers that may be required to work with, or around the contractor/s during the normal course of their duties, members of the public, others at the place of work any other infrastructure or aspects of the worksite.

ORGANISATION'S RESPONSIBILITIES

The Organisation has a duty to ensure, so far as reasonably practicable, the health, safety and welfare at work of all its workers. In particular, it is responsible to ensure:

- That contractors are able to provide evidence of their safety management arrangements for all work to be undertaken by them, acknowledging that any unsafe work will be stopped until it is resolved to the Organisation's satisfaction
- All contractual arrangements to engage contractors stipulates that safety performance is a condition of engagement and that their performance will be monitored and evaluated
- Prospective contractors are provided with sufficient information during the tendering/application process to enable them to respond to any and all identified hazards associated with the scope of work to be performed
- Effective evaluation of any documentation required and provided as prequalification will be used as a selection criteria for the engagement of contractors
- Development and utilisation of a preferred contractor system where possible to ensure that any contractors engaged are selected from this list and therefore already assessed as having appropriate health and safety management practices
- Access to the proposed worksite to allow contractors to undertake specific hazard identification, risk assessment and development of Safe Work Method Statements (SWMS) or equivalent safety procedures before work commences
- Evaluation of any and all Safe Work Method Statements or safety procedures created by contractors for accuracy and appropriateness
- Implementation of a formal consultation schedule (safety meetings and feedback opportunities)
- Communication of the safety requirements and expectations of the Organisation's contractors to the site or project managers, contract managers and/or site superintendents
- That an appropriate corrective action plan is developed and issued to the contractor, or their representative, whenever contractor safety issues are raised on site
- That any work activity or unsafe work practice undertaken by the contractor, or their representative, is ceased immediately if any individual is placed at an immediate risk. The work activity will not resume until the issue is resolved.

CONTRACTOR'S RESPONSIBILITIES

The Contractor and/or sub-contractor must:

- Carry out a site safety assessment in relation to all proposed works
- Undertake all contracted works safely and manage the risk of harm to persons or property
- Ensure that all statutory requirements that require a person to be authorised, licensed, supervised or to have prescribed qualifications or experience are met and be able to produce evidence of the same to the principal contractor if requested, prior to the contractors (or sub-contractors) work commencing
- Ensure that all statutory requirements for the licensing, approvals and/or authorisation of any plant, substance, design or work (or class of work) are met and be able to produce evidence of the same to the head contractor if requested prior to the contractors (or sub-contractors) work commencing
- Develop, implement and maintain a suitable and appropriate emergency management procedures relevant to the proposed contracted works
- If requested by the head contractor (principal), produce evidence of any approvals including any authorisations, licences, prescribed qualifications or experience, or any other information relevant to health and safety (as the case may be) to the satisfaction of

the head contractor (principal) before the contractor or any sub-contractor commences any works
- Generally, comply with the requirements of all safety legislation (or any other legislation that may apply).

WORKER RESPONSIBILITIES

When managing or supervising contractors you are responsible to ensure that you:
- Are familiar with the contents of the contractor's safety management plan
- Undertake monitoring activities as per the agreed schedule
- Contractors maintain their inspection and review schedules
- Report any safety observations to management
- Take immediate action to halt any work being undertaken by contractors that is unsafe and poses an immediate threat to the safety and wellbeing of any persons
- Provide an evaluation of the contractor's safety performance to management at the conclusion of the contracted works
- Demonstrate positive safety behaviours and compliance with the organisation's safety arrangements and instructions.

MOTOR VEHICLES

INTRODUCTION

Operating motor vehicles is a normal part of the Organisation's activities.

Where travelling in the course of duties, the motor vehicle is considered to be a workplace and the Organisation recognises it has health and safety obligations in respect of this.

Risks associated with operating a motor vehicle in the workplace will be addressed via a risk management approach.

IDENTIFYING MOTOR VEHICLE HAZARDS

Motor vehicle hazards can be identified by:
- Reviewing the tasks associated with motor vehicles
- Observing how workers perform their tasks
- Reviewing any documentation regarding use that is provided by the motor vehicle manufacturer or that is otherwise available
- Checking workplace specific documentation regarding the motor vehicle, for example pre-start checklists
- Consulting with the workers carrying out the tasks.

ASSESSING MOTOR VEHICLE HAZARDS

As part of the risk management approach, the Organisation has an obligation to ensure that any motor vehicle operations that pose a risk of injury to workers are assessed to determine the seriousness of these hazards.

In assessing risks arising from motor vehicles, the following factors should be taken into account:
- The size, type and condition of motor vehicles in use
- The licensing requirements for motor vehicle use
- The distances and recommended driving times of trips
- Loading and restraining of loads
- Road and traffic conditions

- Services and amenities on route for refuelling, rest breaks, breakdowns and emergencies.

In addition, any legislative requirements regarding the use of the motor vehicle (including prescribed work, rest, driver fatigue and work diary requirements) will be considered.

CONTROLLING MOTOR VEHICLE RISKS

The Organisation will ensure, as far as reasonably practicable, that the risks associated with motor vehicles in the workplace are controlled. The process of controlling motor vehicle risks will be determined in consultation with the workers who are required to carry out the task.

Only authorised persons will be permitted to operate the Organisation's motor vehicles. The Organisation will put in place systems to ensure that authorised persons are appropriately licensed to drive such motor vehicles, and that the motor vehicles being driven are registered and insured in accordance with the relevant legislation. Photocopies or other records of these checks will be retained.

In the event that motor vehicle operations have been assessed as a risk, the Organisation will:
- Comply with any legislative requirements relating to the use or operation of motor vehicles, for example by scheduling trips to ensure that prescribed work, rest, driver fatigue and work diary requirements are adhered to and ensuring workers have the appropriate licences, certificates and training to operate the motor vehicle. Details of this will be recorded in the **Skills Matrix**
- Ensure that workers are aware of and adhere to trip schedules
- Ensure that the motor vehicle is appropriate for the task
- Ensure that drivers are familiar with the motor vehicle they are required to operate and the safe operation of this
- Ensure that the motor vehicle is inspected, tested and maintained in accordance with the manufacturer's requirements
- Provide mechanical aids where possible to reduce manual handling tasks associated with motor vehicle operations, or otherwise train workers on appropriate manual handling techniques (in particular when loading/unloading the vehicle) and safe operating loads
- Provide instruction and training to workers on this policy and associated procedures.

OFFICE SAFETY

INTRODUCTION

There are a variety of hazards that may arise in an office environment. Controlling these hazards will help to promote the health and safety of workers.

COMMON HAZARDS

i) Desk/workstation ergonomics

A well designed desk/workstation can eliminate health and safety hazards.

The Organisation will ensure, as far as reasonably practicable, that the risks associated with desk/workstation ergonomics in the workplace are controlled. The process of controlling desk/workstation ergonomic risks will be determined in consultation with the workers who are required to utilise a desk/workstation.

Specific areas of focus will include the workers chair, lighting and noise, the position of the screen and the keyboard.

The attached **Appendix 1** outlines specific guidelines for desk/workstation ergonomics. This will be used in conjunction with the **Ergonomics Checklist** to ensure safe workstation setup.

ii) Furniture

The Organisation will ensure, as far as reasonably practicable, the risks associated with office furniture are controlled. This will include ensuring:
* Office furniture is fit for purpose
* Protruding keys are not left in filing cabinet locks
* Filing cabinet and desk drawers are operated using the handles
* Drawers are not left open
* Furniture is arranged so as to avoid trip hazards and obstacles

iii) Passageways and storage

Large objects or groups of people standing around blocking doorways and passageways increases the likelihood of bumps and knocks as vision is blocked and space is tight.

To control these risks, the Organisation will ensure, as far as reasonably practicable, that:
* Doorways and passageways are free of obstruction at all times
* Emergency access and egress are a minimum of 600mm wide and clear of obstruction
* Any area where people walk up and down is sufficiently wide
* Fire extinguishers, fire hydrants, fire alarms and emergency exits are kept free from obstruction
* Items are stored in appropriate areas
* Heavy objects are stored near floor level and appropriate equipment is used to reach objects at height (for example, a stepladder)
* Toxic chemicals are not stored in or near the office.

iv) Floors

The Organisation will ensure, so far as reasonably practicable, that floors do not have objects that can cause slips, trips or falls.

Extension cords and other wires that may cause injury will be secured to the floor or relocated to prevent trip hazards.

Likewise, small items (including litter) left lying on the floor will be removed immediately.

v) Kitchen

Kitchens within the workplace should be kept clean and tidy.

The Organisation will ensure, so far as reasonably practicable, that the following will be regularly cleaned, inspected and maintained:
- microwaves
- fridges
- electric kettles and other electrical equipment
- knives and sharp objects.

WORKING OFFSITE

INTRODUCTION

At times, workers are required to work offsite in settings that are not under the control of the Organisation. This may result in the worker being exposed to additional risks to their health and safety.

Despite not being under its control, the Organisation recognises that offsite work locations may form part of the workplace and therefore health and safety obligations in respect of these sites do apply.

BEFORE WORKING OFFSITE

Where workers are going to work offsite at a location under the control of a host employer, the Organisation will verify with the host employer that all hazards and risks within that setting and associated with the work activity have been identified, assessed and controlled.

This may include:
- Seeking written confirmation/evidence
- Requesting the host employer complete and provide their own documentation or complete the organisation's.

Where workers are working offsite in a setting that is not under the control of a host Organisation (for example, a public domain), a manager or supervisor of the worker is responsible for ensuring that a site risk assessment is completed prior to the work activity commencing. Where it is not practicable for this to occur, the workers will be directed to conduct the risk assessment when they first arrive onsite.

AT THE SITE

Where engaged in offsite work, workers will be directed to comply with any relevant site specific health and safety policies and procedures. In particular, workers will be directed to:
- Report to the site's reception area or designated contact person and announce arrival
- Sign into the site's visitor's attendance log, where required
- Carry/wear any visitor passes whilst on site, as requested
- Attend any site-specific health and safety induction, where required
- Wear/use relevant safety protection clothing issued by the organisation of the site, including any hard hats, personal hearing protection, hi visibility vests, coats, waterproof coats, boots, non-slip soled shoes or goggles.
- Abide by all instructions issued by the site, in particular safety instructions
- Remain on any designated walkways or access paths, and obey any signage on the site

- Report any hazards detected to the site, such as exposed leads or loose railings
- Assess the risk posed by any hazards and determine whether it is safe to continue work. In the event it is not safe to do so, workers will be directed to take necessary steps to prevent an incident occurring and immediately report the hazard to the organisation
- In the event of an emergency, follow the site specific emergency evacuation response plan.

If a health and safety issue or hazard cannot be resolved, the worker will be directed to contact their manager immediately.

WORKING FROM HOME

INTRODUCTION

When workers carry out work at their residential premises (home) for the Organisation, the home is considered to be a workplace and the Organisation recognises that it has health and safety duties in respect of this.

The Organisation must approve all work undertaken at home. The Organisation will only allow for work to be undertaken at home if the hazards associated with the work are identified, assessed and controlled. As such, when approving work to be carried out at home, the Organisation will specify the following:

- The tasks to be performed
- The hours of work
- The specific location within the home where work will be carried out
- The furniture and equipment required to carry out the work.

Based on the above information, risks associated with working at home will be addressed via a risk management approach.

The policies and procedures detailed in this Health and Safety Manual detail how the Organisation manages hazards and risks in the workplace, including those hazards and risks associated with working at home.

IDENTIFYING HAZARDS ASSOCIATED WITH WORKING AT HOME

When working at home, hazards can be identified by:
- Completing the Working from Home Checklist
- Reviewing the tasks associated with working from home
- Observing how workers perform their tasks
- Consulting with relevant workers.

When identifying hazards associated with working at home, the Organisation will consider whether the following hazards are present.

i)   Office safety

There are a variety of hazards that may arise in an office environment which may also be present when working at home.

ii)   **Drugs and alcohol**

The misuse of drugs or alcohol by workers can affect their health and safety, as well as that of others.

iii)   **Remote/Isolated Work**

When working at home, the worker may be working in a remote or isolated environment. Remote / isolated workers can face higher levels of exposure to hazards than workers in a controlled environment. In addition, remote/isolated workers may not have the same access to support and emergency services.

iv)   **Manual handling**

Manual handling describes any work or task involving an action to lift, lower, push, pull, hold, carry, move or restrain any animate or inanimate object.

Some manual handling tasks are hazardous and may cause musculoskeletal disorders. Manual handling injuries are the most common type of workplace injuries across Australia and may occur when working at home.

ASSESSING HAZARDS ASSOCIATED WITH WORKING AT HOME

As part of the risk management approach, the Organisation has an obligation to ensure that any hazards which pose a risk of injury to workers when working at home, are assessed to determine the seriousness of these hazards.

CONTROLLING HAZARDS ASSOCIATED WITH WORKING AT HOME

The Organisation will ensure, as far as reasonably practicable, that the risks associated with working at home are controlled. The process of controlling such risks will be determined in consultation with the workers who are required to work at home.

Control measures can be identified by referring to the following policies detailed within the Health and Safety Manual:
*   Office safety policy
*   Drugs and Alcohol Policy
*   Remote/isolated Work Policy
*   Manual handling policy.

FIRST AID

The Organisation will ensure that workers who are working at home have access to a first aid kit and a trained first aid officer. Details of any workplace injury or illness are to be recorded on the **First Aid Treatment Log/Register of Injuries** and the worker's manager is to be notified as soon as reasonably practicable.

CONSULTATION

The Organisation is committed to providing all workers with the opportunity to express their views and contribute to the resolution of health and safety issues that affect them.

As such the Organisation will consider the use of email and phone calls as a suitable medium for consulting with workers who are working from home.

EMERGENCY PROCEDURES

The Organisation is committed to establishing and maintaining procedures to control emergency situations that could adversely affect workers, including workers who are working at home.

The emergency plans detailed in the Emergency Procedures Policy apply to those workers who are working at home. Furthermore, emergency evacuation exercises will be conducted annually to test the emergency procedures.

Where working at home and affected by an emergency, an **Incident Report Form** is to be completed and the worker's manager is to be notified as soon as reasonably practicable.

WORKPLACE INSPECTIONS

The Organisation will conduct inspections as part of the ongoing management of hazards in the workplace.

When the home is first used as a workplace, the worker will undertake an inspection using the **Working at Home Checklist** and the **Permanent Worksite Inspection Checklist**. Inspections will continue to be undertaken by the worker at least once every six months. Completed checklists are to be provided to the workers manager.

PLANT AND EQUIPMENT

INTRODUCTION

The plant is any machinery, equipment, appliance, implement or tool and any component or fitting used within the workplace.

Plant is machinery that processes material by way of a mechanical action which:
* Cuts, drills, punches or grinds
* Presses forms, hammers, joins, or molds material
* Combines, mixes, sorts, packages, assembles, knits or weaves material.

Plant also includes lifts, cranes, tractors, earth moving equipment, pressure equipment, hoists, powered mobile plant, plant that lifts or moves people or materials, chisels, chainsaws, photocopiers, desks, filing cabinets and temporary access equipment.

Risks associated with plant and equipment in the workplace will be addressed via a risk management approach.

IDENTIFYING PLANT AND EQUIPMENT HAZARDS

Hazard means the potential to cause injury or illness. Examples of potential harm that plant or associated systems of work may cause to people at work include, but are not limited to:
* Injury from entanglement
* Crushing by falling or moving objects, or plant tipping over
* Crushing from people falling off or under plant
* Cutting or piercing due to sharp or flying objects
* Burns (friction, heat, chemical)
* Injury from high-pressure fluids
* Injury from electricity

- Injury from explosion
- Slips trips and falls
- Suffocation
- Ergonomic requirements
- Dust, vibration, noise, or radiation.

ASSESSING PLANT AND EQUIPMENT HAZARDS

As part of the risk management approach, the Organisation has an obligation to ensure that any plant or equipment that may pose a risk of injury to workers is assessed to determine the seriousness of these hazards.

When assessing potential risks and hazards associated with specific plant and equipment considerations should be given to the following throughout the life of the plant:
- Design and construction
- Installation or erection and positioning plant in the workplace
- Commissioning and operation
- Electrical, radiation and thermal energy
- Emergency procedures
- Hazardous substances and dangerous goods
- Machine guarding for plant with moving parts
- Maintenance, repairs, servicing and cleaning requirements
- Manual handling issues
- Noise and vibration
- Personal Protective Equipment requirements
- Work environment including lighting, ventilation, interaction with others
- Safe work procedures and auditing
- Decommissioning, demolition and disposal of plant
- The relevant Australian and international standards.

CONTROLLING PLANT AND EQUIPMENT HAZARDS

The Organisation will ensure, as far as reasonably practicable, that the risks associated with plant and equipment are controlled from purchase through to disposal.

i)   Installation, Erection and Commissioning

Commissioning is a process of verification. This involves an extensive check carried out during the trial phase, prior to the plant being accepted for use. It ensures that the plant performs according to the design criteria and is a process, agreed to by the manufacturer or supplier. The extent and complexity of the commissioning will vary between items of plant.

Plant installation, erection and commissioning must be performed by a competent person who has access to any necessary health and safety information, including any instructions from the designer or manufacturer.

Commissioning methods should:
- Be in accordance with the manufacturer's/supplier's specifications
- Not impose stresses which exceed the limitations of design capabilities include tests to ensure that the plant will perform to its design specifications
- Include typical maintenance checks used by the operator and service personnel
- Be documented

- Ensure the location is suitable for the type of plant and provide sufficient clear space for the plant to be operated, maintained and repaired safely.

The results of the commissioning should include:
- Information about any problems identified during commissioning that suggest the plant cannot be operated safely
- Confirmation that the plant will perform the task for which it has been purchased.
- Specified High Risk Plant needs to be assessed if there is a requirement for the plant to be registered.

ii) Usage and Competency

The Organisation may control a wide variety of plant and equipment in the workplace with workers performing a range of activities and tasks with this equipment. To ensure these activities are conducted in a safe manner, the following processes should be adopted:
- Workers must only use plant when it is capable of performing safely within the design criteria and manufacturer's instructions
- Workers are to be appropriately trained to use/operate the plant and equipment in a safe manner
- Specific work instructions will be developed for the operation of each piece of plant and equipment
- Maintenance and manufacturer's manuals will be kept for all relevant plant and equipment
- appropriate information that states the use for which the plant or equipment has been designed and tested and the conditions that must be followed to ensure the safe use of that plant, will be made available to workers
- Plant and plant equipment is to be used and maintained according to manufacturer's guidelines, inspected and checked for any faults
- Items of heavy plant and machinery need to be checked regularly and recorded in a logbook (a daily pre-start checklist is required)
- Specific inspection checklists may need to be designed for items of plant, such as overhead cranes
- Any incident associated with plant or equipment will be reported to the person's supervisors and they are required to complete an Incident Report Form
- workers are to be advised of the reporting requirements through conducting a toolbox talk
- Supervisors are to regularly check if the plant is being operated correctly.

Some plant and equipment and their use and operation are considered to be high risk work and as such any person who operates or uses the plant or equipment must hold a current National Certificate of Competency or recognised equivalent. The Organisation will maintain a register of licenced operators. Examples of high risk work include:
- Scaffolding
- Dogging and rigging
- Crane and hoist operation (tower cranes, self-erecting tower crane, derrick crane, portal boom cranes, bridge and gantry crane, vehicle loading crane, non-slewing mobile crane, slewing mobile cranes, materials hoist, personnel and materials hoist, boom-type elevating work platform, vehicle-mounted concrete placing boom)
- Forklift operation
- Pressure equipment operation (boilers, turbine, reciprocating steam engine operation)
- Load-shifting equipment (front-end loader/backhoe, front-end loader – skid steer type, excavator)

- Formwork
- Explosive-powered tools
- Operation of motor vehicles requiring the relevant driver's licence.

iii) Modification of plant

As part of the risk management approach, the Organisation will consider all safety issues when considering any alterations to plant and equipment, by:
- Consulting with the designer and manufacturer
- Where the original designer or manufacturer cannot be contacted, the alterations will be carried out by a competent person in accordance with the relevant technical standards. (A competent person is one who has acquired through training, qualification or experience the knowledge and skills to carry out the task)

The Organisation will, so far as is reasonably practicable:
- Ensure that the design and construction of the plant is such that persons who use the plant properly are not, in doing so, exposed to risks to their health and safety
- Ensure that adequate information is supplied about any dangers associated with the plant and about conditions necessary to ensure that persons using the plant properly are not exposed to risk to their health and safety.
- Modifications to protective systems, such as drilling holes or welding, may destroy the integrity of the protective structure. Modifications will not be undertaken unless they have been assessed and specified by a competent person.

iv) Decommissioning and Disposal

When decommissioning and planning for the disposal of plant, the Organisation will:
- Identify and control hazards involved in the process of decommissioning and dismantling the plant
- Dismantle plant in accordance with the designer's and manufacturer's instructions if available
- If re-selling, ensure that the plant is safe to load, transport, unload and store. Any available information relating to the plant design, registration, installation, operation and maintenance will be provided with the plant
- If scrapping, ensure that the plant is safe to load, transport, unload and dispose of /or
- Inform the receiver of the scrap or spare parts (in writing) that they are not to be used as a plant in their present form.

ELECTRICAL SAFETY

INTRODUCTION

Electrical risks are risks of death, electric shock or other injury caused directly or indirectly by electricity and may include:
- Electric shock causing injury or death
- Arcing, explosion or fire causing burns
- Toxic gases from burning and arcing associated with electrical equipment
- Falls from ladders, scaffolds or other elevated work platforms after contact with electricity
- Fire resulting from an electrical fault.

IDENTIFYING THE RISK

The Organisation will consult with workers to identify electrical hazards arising from electrical equipment or installations. The following will be considered to assist in the identification of electrical risk:

- The design, construction, installation, maintenance and testing of electrical equipment or electrical installations
- Inadequate or inactive electrical protection, for example no or damaged safety switches
- Where and how electrical equipment is used, for example electrical equipment may be at a greater risk of damage if used outdoors or in a factory or workshop environment
- Electrical equipment being used in an area in which the atmosphere presents a risk to health and safety from fire or explosion, for example using grinders in areas where flammable fumes may be present
- Type of electrical equipment, for example 'plugin' electrical equipment that is moved from site to site, including extension leads, are particularly liable to damage
- The age and condition of electrical equipment and electrical installations
- Work carried out on or near electrical equipment or electrical installations such as electric overhead lines or underground electric services
- Reviewing incident reports.

ASSESSING THE RISK

The Organisation will consult with workers to assess the risk associated with electrical hazards considering the following:

- The conditions under which the electrical equipment is used, for example wet conditions outdoors or at construction sites
- Work practices and procedures, for example using electrical equipment in flammable atmospheres
- The capability, skill and experience of relevant workers.

CONTROLLING THE RISK

The Organisation will consult with workers to determine control actions for eliminating or minimising electrical risks.

Where the hazard cannot be eliminated, for example by using hand tools in place of power tools in flammable atmospheres, or de-energising equipment and circuits prior to conducting work, the Organisation will minimise the risk associated with electrical equipment and installations considering the following:

- Replacing a power tool that is plugged into mains electricity with an extra-low voltage battery-operated tool
- Using safety switches (portable or fixed) to minimise the risk, for example installing residual current devices to reduce the risk of receiving a fatal electric shock
- Administrative controls and safe work practices, for example determining electrical and gas lines prior to the use of tools to penetrate walls, floors and ceilings, use of permits and warning signs.

Unsafe electrical equipment must be disconnected or isolated from its electricity supply. It must not be reconnected unless it is repaired by a competent person or tests by a competent person have confirmed it is safe to use. Alternatively, it could be replaced or permanently removed from use.

Unsafe electrical equipment should be labelled indicating it is unsafe and must not be used. This is to prevent inadvertent use before the electrical equipment can be tested, repaired or replaced.

Serious injuries and fatalities may be prevented by the use of properly installed and maintained residual current devices (RCDs), commonly referred to as 'safety switches'. An RCD is an electrical safety device designed to immediately switch off the supply of electricity when electricity 'leaking' to earth is detected at harmful levels. RCDs offer high levels of personal protection from electric shock.

ELECTRICAL EQUIPMENT TESTING AND TAGGING

Electrical equipment used in lower-risk operating environments does not require inspection and testing or tagging if connected to a fixed safety switch. However, where electrical equipment is:

- Supplied with electricity through an electrical socket outlet ('plugin' equipment), and
- Used in an environment in which its normal use exposes the equipment to operating conditions that are likely to result in damage to the equipment or a reduction in its expected lifespan, for example moisture, heat, vibration, mechanical damage, corrosive chemicals or dust
- The Organisation will ensure that the electrical equipment is regularly inspected and tested by a competent person as per the timings set out below.

Portable electrical equipment: appliances, flexible cords, cord extension sets, portable socket outlet assemblies (eg powerboards), generators, inverters		Residual Current Devices (Safety Switches)			
		Push button test by user		Operating time/ current test	
Environment	Portable electrical equipment	Fixed	Portable	Fixed	Portable
Construction work	3 months	monthly	daily	12 months	3 months
Manufacturing work: factories, workshops, places of manufacture, assembly, maintenance or fabrication.	6 months	6 months	N/A	12 months	N/A
Service work: environments where the equipment or flexible cord is subject to flexing in normal use OR is in a hostile environment.	12 months	6 months	3 months	12 months	12 months
Residential type areas: hotels, residential institutions, motels, boarding houses, halls, hostels, accommodation houses, and the like	2 years	6 Months	6 months	2 years	2 years
Office work: environments where the equipment or cord is NOT subject to flexing in normal use and is NOT open to abuse and is NOT in a hostile environment.	5 yearly	6 months	3 months	2 years	2 years
Rural industry work (all plug in equipment)	visual examination before each use	N/A	N/A	N/A	N/A
Commercial cleaning equipment	6 months	daily	N/A	6 months	N/A

WORKING AT HEIGHTS

INTRODUCTION

Falls are a major cause of death and serious injury in Australian workplaces. Fall hazards are found in many workplaces where work is carried out at heights (for example, stacking shelves, working on a roof, or unloading a large truck). Fall hazards may also arise at ground level, for example trenches or service pits. Predominantly, fall hazards pose a risk to the individual worker, however hazards may also arise for workers on ground level where the risk of falling objects is a concern.

Any Organisation performing work from heights using a harness - fall arrest systems, Elevated Work Platforms, Scissor Lifts or Man Cage (Forklift) - MUST have a rescue plan in place and all workers performing tasks must be trained in the plan.

Risks associated with falls in the workplace will be addressed via a risk management approach.

IDENTIFYING WORKING AT HEIGHTS HAZARDS

The Organisation, in consultation with workers, will identify working at heights risks in the workplace by:
- Reviewing tasks that are carried out, including those that are carried out:
  o on plant or structures at an elevated level or to gain access to an elevated level
  o on or in the vicinity of an opening, void or fragile surface through which a person could fall (for example, cement sheeting roofs, rusty metal roofs, fibreglass sheeting roofs and skylights)
  o on or in the vicinity of an edge over which a person could fall
  o on or in the vicinity of a slippery, sloping or unstable surface
  o on or in areas where there is restricted and or limited access
  o on any structure or plant, including those being constructed, installed, demolished, dismantled, inspected, tested, repaired or cleaned
- Observing how workers perform their tasks
- Reviewing plant and equipment in the workplace and any documentation regarding the use of fall prevention, fall arrest and Personal Protective Equipment provided by the equipment manufacturer or that is otherwise available
- Checking workplace specific documentation regarding the work area or task
- Consulting with the workers carrying out the tasks
- Considering the risk of falling objects when working at heights.

ASSESSING WORKING AT HEIGHTS RISKS

When assessing the risks arising from working at heights, the Organisation will consider the following:
- The design and layout of elevated work areas, including the distance of a potential fall
- The number and movement of all people at the workplace
- The adequacy of inspection and maintenance of plant and equipment (for example, scaffolding)
- The adequacy of lighting for clear vision
- The nature of the work area and the potential impact of weather conditions, including rain, wind, extreme heat or cold

Appendix

- The suitability of worker footwear and clothing for nature and location of work being performed
- The suitability and condition of any plant or equipment (for example, ladders) used to access heights or whilst working at heights, including where and how they are being used
- The level of knowledge of workers working at heights, and any training required to allow the worker to perform the task safely, particularly for young, new or inexperienced workers
- The adequacy of procedures for all potential emergency situations, and any amendments that may be required for workers working at heights:
- The proximity of Overhead Power Lines and the movement of workers, plant and equipment around the work site: and
- Work practices where goods, materials and tools must be carried whilst ascending or descending stairs ramps and walkways

In addition, the Organisation will consider the proximity of workers to elevated working areas (for example, loading docks) where loads are placed, and areas where work is carried out above people, to assess the risks associated with falling objects.

CONTROLLING WORKING AT HEIGHTS RISKS

The Organisation will ensure, as far as reasonably practicable, that the risks of falls and falling objects associated with working at heights are controlled. The process of controlling these risks will be determined in consultation with workers.

In the event that falls and falling objects have been assessed as a risk, the Organisation will wherever practicable eliminate the need to work at heights by carrying out work on the ground or on a permanent structure that complies with legislative requirements.

Where the above controls are not practicable, the Organisation will do the following where necessary and reasonably practicable:
- Provide and maintain fall prevention devices (for example, guard rails)
- Provide a work positioning system (for example, an industrial rope access system)
- Provide a fall-arrest system, for example a harness
- Provide appropriate PPE (for example, gloves and footwear)
- Ensure that workers required to work at heights have any required licenses/certificates
- Provide task specific training to workers required to work at heights, for example on the use of fall arrest devices, elevated work platforms or scaffolds.

SUN SAFETY

INTRODUCTION

Australia has one of the highest rates of skin cancer in the world. Despite being an almost entirely preventable disease at least two in every three Australians will develop skin cancer before they reach the age of 70. Of all new cancers diagnosed in Australia each year, 80 percent are skin cancers.
Workers who work outdoors for all or part of the day have a higher than average risk of skin cancer. This is because ultraviolet radiation in sunlight or 'solar UVR' is a known carcinogen.

All skin types can be damaged by exposure to solar UVR. Damage is permanent and irreversible and increases with each exposure.

As part of the risk management approach, the Organisation has an obligation to ensure that any risks associated with exposure to solar UVR are eliminated or controlled. Through adopting a hierarchy of controls and as far as reasonably practicable, the Organisation will eliminate or minimise the risks from exposure to solar UVR for outdoor workers.

ORGANISATIONS RESPONSIBILITIES

The Organisation will:
- Assess the risks in consultation with workers to identify those workers who have a high risk of exposure to solar UVR and work situations where exposure to solar UVR occurs
- Minimise, so far as reasonably practicable, workers' exposure to solar UVR by consulting with workers and ensuring workers use sun protection control measures during sun protection times and at all times when working outdoors for extended periods
- Actively supervise outdoor workers and monitor their use of sun protection control measures
- Ensure injury reporting procedures are followed when an incident of sunburn or excessive exposure to solar UVR occurs in the workplace
- Provide training to workers to enable them to work safely in the sun
- Ensure training is provided as part of induction for new workers
- Ensure workers are provided with information to effectively examine their own skin
- Ensure managers and supervisors act as positive role models
- Promote the use of sun protection control measures 'off the job'
- Recognise that a combination of sun protection control measures provides the best protection to workers from exposure to solar UVR.

CONTROL MEASURES

In accordance with the Risk Management approach and using the hierarchy of controls, where possible, the Organisation will:
- Provide shaded areas or temporary shade.
- Encourage workers to move jobs to shaded areas.
- Modify reflective surfaces.
- Identify and minimise contact with photosensitising substances.
- Provide indoor areas or shaded outdoor areas for rest and meal breaks.
- Schedule outdoor work tasks to occur when levels of solar UVR are less intense e.g. Earlier in the morning or later in the afternoon.
- Schedule indoor and shaded work tasks to occur when levels of solar UVR are strongest eg in the middle part of the day.
- Encourage workers to rotate between indoor, shaded and outdoor tasks to avoid exposure to solar UVR for long periods of time.
- Provide personal protective equipment (PPE), including:
- Sun protective work clothing such as long-sleeved shirts with a collar and trousers or knee-length shorts
- Sun protective hats covering the face, head, ears and neck
- Sunglasses meeting Australian Standards, and
- Broad-spectrum, SPF 30 or higher, water resistant sunscreen.

HEAT STRESS

WORKING SAFELY IN HOT CONDITIONS

The Worker Induction Handbook contains a Procedure for Sun Safety and this information supports that procedure as heat stress may affect people during the summer months and in some workplaces, it can be an issue all year around.

Heat stress is the total heat burden the body is subjected to by both internal and external factors. The body must balance the heat inputs to the body, heat generated in the body and heat coming out of the body.

Risks associated with heat stress in the workplace will be addressed via a risk management approach.

IDENTIFYING HEAT STRESS HAZARDS

While some hazards associated with heat stress are well understood there may be factors you were not aware of. Some individuals will be more prone to heat stress if they are medically unfit, on certain medications, overweight, have heart disease, are pregnant, abuse alcohol, or are not acclimatised to the conditions. Heed medical advice.

Even for workers that are well accustomed to working in the heat, time away from work will change the body's normal response. Acclimatisation is lost to some degree after 3 days away from work and entirely lost after four weeks away. Re-acclimatisation takes 7 – 14 days after returning to this type of work and exposure.

If the body can't balance heat inputs heat stress may lead to heat illness, a physical response designed to reduce your body temperature.

Types of heat illness include:
*   **Discomfort** - flushed skin, increased sweating, heat rashes (prickly heat)
*   **Mild heat illness** - feeling tired weak or dizzy, cramps, reduced work capacity, reduced attention span, irritability
*   **Heat exhaustion** - fainting, headache, low blood pressure, nausea, clammy pale or flushed skin, normal to high body temperature (up to 39C)
*   **Heat stroke** - irritability, confusion, speech problems, hot dry skin, convulsions, unconsciousness, body temperature above 40C, cardiac arrest – potentially fatal

Heat stress causes increased blood flow to the skin which allows the release of heat. Blood is diverted to the muscles if physical work is being performed resulting in a lower release of heat through the skin.

CONTROLLING THE HAZARDS

Workers must be protected from extremes of heat and there is a recommended order of controls to eliminate or reduce the risk of harm often a combination of controls will be needed and these risks will be determined in consultation with the workers who are required to carry out the task.

i)   Engineering

- Increase air movement with supplementary fans
- Install shade structures to reduce radiant heat
- Install shields or barriers to reduce radiant heat from sources such as hot machinery
- Use mechanical aids to reduce exertion

ii)   Organisation of work

- Reschedule work during the cooler times of the day or year
- Reduce the time spent by individuals by task rotation
- Arrange more workers to do the job
- Ensure easy access to cool drinking water
- Provide additional rest breaks in the shade or indoors

iii)   Personal Protective Equipment

- Broad brimmed hat
- Protective clothing should cover to at least elbows and knees
- Sunscreen
- Sunglasses

PERSONAL PROTECTIVE EQUIPMENT (PPE)

INTRODUCTION

Exposure and injury can be prevented with the use of PPE where preventative measures for a hazard require additional control. Use of PPE is only to be considered when more effective control measures have been ruled out.

Hearing protection, eye protection, skin protection, respiratory protection and other personal protection can be achieved by wearing specific items developed to prevent injury.

Risks associated with PPE in the workplace will be addressed via a risk management approach.

ORGANISATION'S RESPONSIBILITIES

The Organisation shall:
- Ensure they supply suitable PPE and protective clothing
- That PPE and protective clothing meets relevant legislative, Australian Standard and/or industry requirements or guidelines
- Ensure that information and training is provided in the correct use, wear and maintenance of PPE and protective clothing supplied
- Ensure tasks are assessed to determine the correct level of PPE required
- Ensure that PPE and protective clothing being used are in an appropriate condition for the works being performed
- Replace damaged or worn PPE and protective clothing
- Ensure their workers wear and use such items supplied to them.

Appendix

WORKER RESPONSIBILITIES

Workers have a responsibility to:
* Wear and use PPE and protective clothing provided as instructed
* Maintain and care for the PPE and protective clothing supplied
* Report damaged or worn PPE to your manager.

DETERMINATION OF PPE AND PROTECTIVE CLOTHING

Determination of whether PPE and/or specific protective clothing are required will be based on a risk assessment of a hazard or task and, where relevant:
* The Information contained in the SDS for chemicals and dangerous goods
* Operating procedures for the plant,
* SWMS, and
* Safe operating or work procedures.

SELECTION OF PPE AND PROTECTIVE CLOTHING

All PPE selected shall conform to the appropriate legislative, Australian Standard and/or industry requirements or guidelines.

PPE supplied by the Organisation remains the property of the Organisation.

Before any PPE is used it should be inspected to ensure:
* A good fit for the user
* It is appropriate for the task and will protect the user from the hazards it is intended to control
* It does not introduce any new hazards
* Is in good condition
* The user understands the correct usage of the equipment.

If there are any defects or deficiencies found with the PPE after inspection it must be taken out of service immediately and reported to the manager.

New products are continually being developed and made available this may mean an item that has been in use may be superseded and no longer available.

If new equipment requires selection, the most effective PPE should be chosen according to the risk assessment or SDS information.

PROTECTION

Where defined by signage on the plant, entrances to buildings/rooms or work sites all identified PPE must be worn.

DESK/WORKSTATION ERGONOMICS

In the event that desk/workstation ergonomics have been identified as a risk, the Organisation should implement the below control measures.

i)   Chair

Seat height should be adjusted so the worker's feet rest firmly on the floor at a right angle and take the weight through the feet. Thighs should be fully supported except for a two finger width space behind the knee. Thighs should be parallel or slightly inclined towards the floor. The worker should maintain a relaxed posture where the:

- Shoulders are relaxed
- Elbows are by their side
- Forearms and hands are parallel to the ground, with an angle of approximately 90 degrees at the elbow
- Wrists are not bent or cocked when using the keyboard
- Seat is at a comfortable distance from the keys, approximately the length of a forearm away
- Backrest is adjusted to enable the worker to sit upright for typing.

ii)   Computer screens

The top of the screen should be approximately at eye level and about 35 -70cm from the worker's eyes.

iii)   Keyboard

The worker should be able to maintain the recommended seating position when using the keyboard. A fixed keyboard surface that is too high will require the worker to raise the seat height to attain the correct position. A suitable footrest should be used to support their feet in this instance.

The keyboard should be placed 6-7cm from the edge of the desk to allow the workers forearm/wrist to rest when not typing.

iv)   Mouse

Ensure there is no overreaching to the mouse and that the worker can manipulate the mouse with both hands. Workers should also be educated on the user 'shortcut' keys on the keyboard.

v)   Documents

The document and screen should be placed the same distance from the worker's eyes. A document holder should be provided to allow the worker to place the documents in the most convenient position.

Documents should be placed:
- On a level position beside the screen when the keyboards is in a central position
- Directly below the screen just above the keyboard.

vi)   Glare

Altering the angle of the worker's screen by a maximum of 5 degrees may overcome problems with glare and reflection.

Appendix

Generally, the best position for the screen is at right angles (side on) to the windows. Where this is not possible, reflection and glare can be controlled by blinds.

vii) Breaks

When typing, workers should take short, frequent breaks of 30-60 seconds. They should relax their hands away from the keyboard.

viii) Layout

Ensure all frequently used items are within easy reach and that there is sufficient space for large documents, completed work or writing.

Ensure the workstation is designed to prevent undue twisting of the neck or trunk.

REGISTER OF NOTIFIABLE INCIDENT

Employers are required to keep a register of Notifiable Incidents that are readily accessible in the workplace (Under Section 63 of the Workplace Injury Management and Workers Compensation Act 1998). The manager of any mine or quarry, or the occupier of any factory, workshop, office or shop is responsible for this register of injuries.

Requirements of Injury and Illness Registration

- Employers must keep a **Register of Injuries** at each workplace for workers to record any workplace injury or illness
- The register of injuries may be kept in electronic form only if the employer provides education, training and facilities to ensure that workers are able to access the register.
- An injured worker (or someone acting on their behalf) must notify the employer in writing, or verbally, of any work-related injury or illness as soon as possible after an injury has happened
- Employers need to provide written confirmation to the injured worker that they received notification of the injury or illness
- Employers need to provide a signed and dated copy of the state's Incident Form to the injured or ill worker

Information in relation to Work Health and Safety Laws

If you are responsible under the Work Health and Safety (WHS) laws for workers other than employees, for example contractors, you may not be required under workers compensation laws to record injuries in your register of injuries. However, you may find it helpful to do so. If you wish to include details of all injuries in the one place you should add space in the template to indicate whether or not the person is an employee for workers compensation purposes.

WHS INDUCTION CHECKLIST - WORKSITE

This induction checklist must accompany the new employee during the site induction process.

Inductee details

Surname:	First name(s):

Please select which employment status represents the type of inductee

○ **Administration**   ○ **Staff Member**   ○ **Subcontractor**   ○ **Contractor**

Department assigned to:
Proposed Job Title:
Line Manager:
Inductor:
Date Commenced:

Inductee Item Checklist

Inductor and Worker to initial when each item is completed			Inductor	Worker
Qualifications established and recorded *Check and copy all licenses, Certificates of Competency, Verification of Competency Cards etc. required to carry out tasks*	○ **Yes**	○ **N/A**		
Completed Company WHS Induction	○ **Yes**	○ **N/A**		
Shown the location of first aid facilities and first aid attendants	○ **Yes**			
Shown the fire extinguisher location in work area	○ **Yes**			
Site Evacuation Procedures explained Assembly Point and Evacuation Route Emergency Wardens and their locations Provision for Offsite emergencies	○ **Yes**			
Shown kitchen amenities, toilets and drinking water	○ **Yes**			
Initial on-the-job training for daily routine	○ **Yes**			
Accident/incident/near miss reporting explained	○ **Yes**			
Site Non-Smoking Policy explained	○ **Yes**			
Site Drug and Alcohol Policy explained	○ **Yes**			

Appendix

Issued protective equipment/safety gear (PPE)	○ **Yes**	○ **N/A**		
Shirt/pants	○ **Yes**	○ **N/A**		
Other:	○ **Yes**	○ **N/A**		
Inductee introduced to:				
Supervisors	○ **Yes**	○ **N/A**		
Administration	○ **Yes**	○ **N/A**		
Initial Introduction to the immediate work environment Site specific hazards and risk assessments explained	○ **Yes**	○ **N/A**		
Induction to relevant procedures (incl SWMS/JSA)	○ **Yes**	○ **N/A**		
Any specialised equipment and training in use	O **Yes**	○ **N/A**		
Hazardous substances locations and procedures (storage, spills, SDS, etc.)	○ **Yes**	○ **N/A**		
Machinery Safety – Significance/use of "Out of Service" and "Danger" tags explained	○ **Yes**	○ **N/A**		
All site procedures and rules including hours of work and security explained	○ **Yes**	○ **N/A**		
Tour of work site provided	○ **Yes**	○ **N/A**		
Site induction card has been issued	○ **Yes**	○ **N/A**		
Health and Safety Handbook issued	○ **Yes**	○ **N/A**		

Declaration

I acknowledge that I, the undersigned, have been advised on all of the above listed items and understand the points discussed. Where appropriate, I also undertake to use and have been instructed in the correct usage of Personal Protective Equipment (PPE). I accept that compliance with safe work practices is a condition of my continued access to the site and also a requirement under the WHS legislation.

The inductor has reiterated the key points of this induction program and I understand the procedures involved.

Workers Name (Please print)	**Signature**	**Date**
Inductor's Name (Please print)	**Signature**	**Date**

ADDITIONAL RESOURCES

The Queensland Incident Investigation Form can be found at
https://www.worksafe.qld.gov.au/__data/assets/pdf_file/0020/82505/incidents_form.pdfv

Please refer to the Workers Compensation Regulation 2016 (www.legislation.nsw.gov.au) for more detailed information.

Further Information

To notify a 'notifiable incident' contact your local regulator.

Jurisdiction	Regulator	Telephone	Website
New South Wales	SafeWork NSW	13 10 50	safework.nsw.gov.au
Victoria	WorkSafe Victoria	1800 136 089	worksafe.vic.gov.au
Queensland	WorkSafe Queensland	1300 369 915	worksafe.qld.gov.au
South Australia	SafeWork SA	1800 777 209	safework.sa.gov.au
Western Australia	WorkSafe WA	1300 307 877	commerce.wa.gov.au/WorkSafe/
Australian Capital Territory	WorkSafe ACT	02 6207 3000	worksafe.act.gov.au/healthsafety
Tasmania	WorkSafe Tasmania	1300 366 322 (Tas) 03 6233 7657 (External)	worksafe.tas.gov.au
Northern Territory	NT WorkSafe	1800 019 115	worksafe.nt.gov.au
Commonwealth	Comcare	1300 366 979	comcare.gov.au

This information sheet has been prepared using the latest information available. No warranties to the suitability of the information for your specific circumstances and disclaims all responsibility and liability for all expenses, losses, damages and costs you might incur as a result of the information being inaccurate or incomplete.

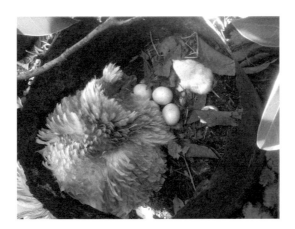

Appendix

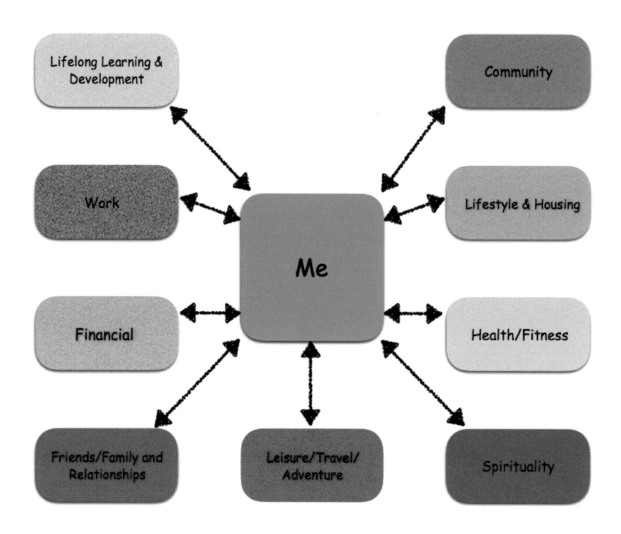

How has your past sculpted your present?

In order to write your life plan there are a few simple things that need to be in order first:

- Set aside a full day to be with yourself to get creative, be in the best possible frame of mind. Decide what location you want to be to write your plan down
- Take everything that you need in order to start and complete the process undisturbed. E.g. pens/paper/music/food/water. Leave behind guilt and electronic devices. Advise family/friends/other necessary acquaintances that you are unavailable for some time
- Check in with your attitude, create a sense of anticipation, expectation, gratitude and openness

Trust the process, listen to your heart and don't worry about getting it all right. Stay focused and see it through to the end. Some sections will be easier than others and that is normal. You can't start your new life if you still have parts missing in it. What you resist persists

- What would you do if money weren't an issue? Give yourself permission to dream big
- What have been the significant moments in your life? Some will be absolutely amazing and some may have left you feeling sad, shameful or guilty.
- How have you become the person you are today? What have been the major influences in your life? E.g. family, relationships, health, fitness, finances, events.
- When you look back on your life what do you immediately think of? E.g. highlights, traumas, beginnings, completions.
- What goals and dreams have come true for you personally? How did you achieve these?
- What failures have happened over your life so far? What were the valuable lessons you've learnt? E.g. learnt to respond not react, sometimes the answer will be "no!", I forgive, it's better to be kind than right.....

Frame every so-called disaster with these words "in 5 years' time will this still matter?"
- What/who has transformed your life for the better and why? What did you gain or give up in order to have this happen?
- What have you learnt about yourself so far? Name the good and the bad. E.g persistent/procrastinator/over eager/people pleaser/don't put myself first....
- What would you change if you could?
- What do you want to experience more of? E.g. physically, mentally, emotionally, spiritually, nutritionally.
- Do you need a wake-up call in order to change some habits or beliefs?
- How often have you just drifted without a clue where you're heading, and then wondered how you ended up here?

When it comes to going after what you want, exhaust all avenues.
- Do you get off track because of confusion, expenses, lost opportunities, pain, regrets?
- Are you honest with yourself: about your current: bank account? physically? mentally? emotionally? spiritually? nutritionally?
- Have you decided where you want to go in life? Are you aiming in the right direction of success?

Live in the question of "what are the infinite possibilities of my life being....(whatever you desire)?"

Recognise the 'law of diminishing intent' says that the longer you delay doing something, the less probability you have of actually doing it. You lose all the emotional energy.
Be flexible with your life plan, it will constantly need tweaking depending on the unforeseeable circumstances beyond your control. E.g. injury to yourself, others or the economy.

Before we start planning for the future, it's really important to take stock of where you are right now. We are looking at the baseline of where we are starting.

Every life plan needs passion and enthusiasm to make it come alive and meaningful to you. Engage every sense, you need to be able to see, hear, smell, taste and feel your goals.

Let's start by looking at what you consider to be your strengths and weaknesses. This will raise some thoughts of what you would like to change.

Life Balance

Strengths

These are positive attributes, tangible and intangible, internal and within your control. Some examples could be:

- I can adjust quickly to environment/situations
- I have a positive attitude to life
- For most occasions I believe in my own abilities
- I'm able to ask for guidance when needed
- I have no financial worries
- I enjoy and have a great work/social/play life
- Academia comes easily when I apply myself
- I embrace the many opportunities to travel
- I'm mostly optimistic
- I have a healthy strong body and enjoy exercising
- I enjoy 'personal quiet time' alone or with company
- I am confident and own my uniqueness and talents
- I know what having financial freedom feels like

Weaknesses

Weaknesses are factors that are within your control that detract from your ability to gain or support a positive attitude. Some examples could be:

- I think nothing is ever good enough: it's either too hot/too cold/too wet/to dark/too early/too tired
- I stress that there is never enough to go around: clothes to wear/money/transport
- My body hurts, I'm often too sore to enjoy life
- Often, I feel better than everyone else: I know better, I find weaknesses in other people/trainers/friends/family/work colleagues
- I always find faults when I ask for advice. I also often criticise or find fault to any solution offered
- I am often a "yes" person. I conform. I don't want to upset anyone. I'll go without. I won't rock the boat. I'll stick to the rule
- I always control situations and become bossy: Do it my way, let me set rules and I expect others to follow regardless
- I don't really like my own company: I can't go or do it on my own, I mostly prefer company
- I don't like to make decisions: I'd rather hurt myself and avoid confrontation, I'll go along with advice even if its detrimental to me
- I manipulate others: I'll only do it if you do, I play on other people's weaknesses, or get sympathy I often play the "poor me"
- I'm materialistic: I consider my clothes/gym gear/car are better – I can prove I'm doing "ok" by what I own...
- I'm too much of a dreamer: I'll be better at this when.....nothing is ever good enough, always whining about something
- I procrastinate: I'll start tomorrow, I always putting off for tomorrow what I could have done today
- I can be a bit of a space cadet: I spend too much time thinking and not enough time doing
- I'm a perfectionist: It's never good enough. I constantly find fault in myself, others or equipment
- I've lost my own identity: It makes me feel important when others need me, but I don't really know what I like any more

- I enjoy shocking people: I'm a thrill seeker, I bet you can't do this....I'm always looking for the shock value in things I do. I'm always striving for uniqueness
- I laugh too much: I'll pretend that I'm ok, I'd rather appear happy than to show the real pain
- I'm always way too busy: There are never enough hours in the day, I'm always governed by a timetable/time line
- I don't deal with rejection very well, I always take things personally

Opportunities

After having a look at your current reality, take some time to think about some of the influences you know you may be facing in the near future of 6-12 months. What are the external positive factors that represent reasons you're likely to succeed in life?
- I have a chance to apply the training I have been doing
- I'm expecting some money to come to me within the next 6 months
- I have a strong supportive family that will help me with a major decision soon
- When I finish my study it will secure my employment contract
- My car will be repaired and I am then free to go on weekend holidays
- I have a mentor who is helping me with my advertising campaign that will launch this October
- My health support group has invited me to do a talk at the community hall in November

Threats

Is there anything that you feel would be an external or negative threat to you that is beyond your control that could hinder your life goals within the near future?
- Work has expanded and I am worried I will lose my secure position within the "family environment"
- A family member is getting sicker and it's possible I will have to "put my life on hold" to care for them
- If the country that I'm traveling to is politically unsteady, I may not be able to get my work visa
- My partner has had a work transfer and we have to relocate
- My bills are mounting up and getting out of control, unless I seek professional help I will soon be having the debt collectors at my door step

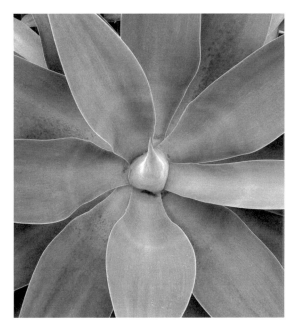

GOALS: WHERE ARE YOU GOING?

Your Personal Mission & Vision Claim

Your personal vision is the driver, motivator and reason for being/doing what makes your heart sing. This is where you dream big and allow the imagination to take wings

Write a sentence or short paragraph, which combine physical, emotional, and logical elements into one exceptional amazing summary that reflects your core purpose, identity, reason, values and main reasons for being who and what your do. Provide a broad, inspirational image of the future you seek to create.

How do you want to be remembered by God, spouse, children, parents, colleagues, and friends? Can you clarify your priorities and live with purpose?

What matters most to you? By being in balance we can give appropriate attention to each area of our life. This can become your vision board, your screen saver or anywhere else you would love to display your true identity.

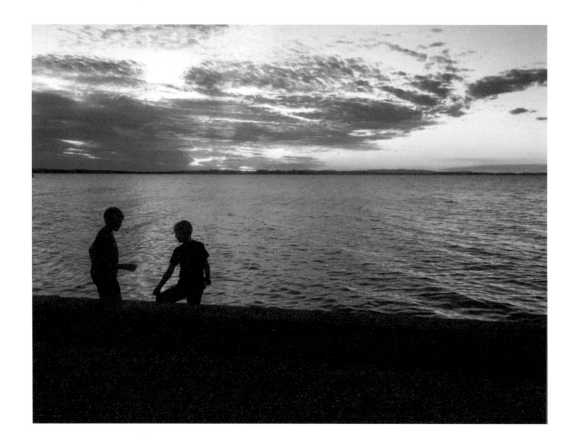

GOALS & OBJECTIVES

Now that you have faced reality it's time to start kicking butt. You can't change what you won't face or own.

Now you know where your life really is, having done your life summary up until this point, you can now set realistic life goals for the next 12 months in a quantifiable, measurable and fun way. You need to be specific here.

Are your goals S.M.A.R.T? Specific, measurable, actionable, realistic, time-bound. Whatever the goal, small daily investments can bring you big results.

What are the infinite possibilities of your life?

We have divided your life into 9 very broad areas. These are guidelines only and if you feel like you would like to change the names or add more areas to your chart then feel totally free to do as you wish.

The areas of your life that you will be setting your goals for fall into the following 9 categories. Prioritise your top 7-10 goals for this year, remembering you want to be able to achieve every single one of them. This time next year you will be rocking it, feeling like a big 'winner' in your own life. Dream big, then break it down into bite size chunks.

- **Friends/Family and Relationships:** E.g. This summer I will join a walking club and meet new friends and I will create new interests
- **Leisure/Travel/Adventure:** E.g. This winter I will book my tickets and accommodation to go snow skiing for 3 weeks
- **Financial:** E.g. This financial year I shall save $5,000 towards my new car
- **Health/Fitness:** E.g. By my birthday I will be able to swim 1km without stopping
- **Spirituality:** E.g. I will deepen my meditation and devotion by doing half an hour twice a day starting today
- **Lifestyle & Housing:** E.g. I will improve my lifestyle and my housing by de-cluttering every cupboard every season
- **Paid Work:** E.g. I will have finished the major project of (....) that I have been working on by June 30th
- **Community:** E.g. I will be helping in the kitchen at a community support group by February
- **Lifelong Learning & Development:** E.g. I will learn to speak French before my European holiday in 3 years' time

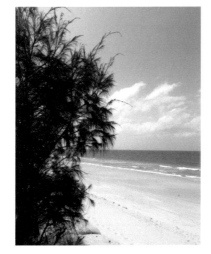

LETS GET INTO ACTION

How can you get from where you are today to where you want to be in the future? Now is the time to clarify specific goals of where you want to be and how you will get there.

- Have the end in mind when you are envisioning the future. Use your imagination, what are the infinite possibilities of everything turning out just fine?
- Here are some questions to ask yourself below that will help you flesh out what is important to you. Enjoy!!

FAMILY & RELATIONSHIPS

Physical
- How can you put yourself first? You can't take care of anyone else if you don't look after yourself
- What are some adventures you would like to go on with friends/family?
- What could you create together as a family?
- How can you nurture your family and friends when they need you? E.g. quality time/gifts/acts of service/physical touch/kind words
- How can you spend more quality time with your children?

Mental
- How can you give yourself permission to make mistakes while you learn? Maybe you can write your thoughts down as it forces you to get close and focused on a more positive outcome?
- How can you effectively praise good behaviour and correct lovingly attention seeking behaviour?
- What is special or a tradition that you value in your family or relationships? How can you make more time to do them?
- How can you respond rather than react to situations? E.g. take a long slow breath as it calms the mind
- What do you need to get rid of that isn't useful, beautiful or joyful?

Emotional
- How can you focus on what matters and let go of the small stuff? E.g. All that truly matters is that you're loved
- As a mum/dad, wife/husband/partner, friend/sibling/relation what could you do in order to experience more joy?
- How can you allow yourself to trust your instincts more each day?
- How can you help your family blossom?
- What are the all the ways you can allow each family member to feel safe about talking about what is near and dear to their heart?
- How could you have less crazy/stressful times?
- How quickly can you find the positives in every story?
- Can you hold space for others to express themselves freely?
- Do you have time to breathe, reflect and act?
- Do you recognise when people need more love? Sometimes it's better to be kind than right
- Do you allow yourself to release emotions? E.g. Crying with someone is more healing than crying alone. Its ok to let your children see you cry
- Do you have an open communication policy? E.g. If a relationship has to be a secret, you shouldn't be in it

- Is everyday a special occasion worth celebrating? E.g. Burn candles, use nice sheets, and wear fancy lingerie.

Spiritual

- Do you make time for your spiritual traditions in your family or relationships?
- Do you have a connection to your God that you feel you can share?
- Can you forgive family and friends?

Nutritional

- What mealtime or dining traditions are in your family or relationships? Do you make time to celebrate them?
- Are you happy with the nutritional circles you are in? E.g. healthy food vs. processed, drugs, addictive behaviour
- Do you eat to sustain your stamina, emotional and mental well-being: Food dictates your mood?

LEISURE & TRAVEL

Physical

- What places or who would you like to visit this year?
- Can you prepare for a holiday, then go with the flow and trust?

Mental

- If you can't travel, can you take adventures in a book or through a movie or even stories told by others?
- Could you learn another language?
- If you could be anywhere, where is the most relaxing Zen space for you to go to?

Emotional

- Would your next holiday be to relax, take an adventure, be with family, or to be by yourself?
- Do you own your own happiness and make it happen?

Spiritual

- If you were to have a spiritual holiday, where would you go?
- Would you discover other spiritual cultures when you travel?

Nutritional

- Are you in need of a detox holiday?

FINANCES & LEGAL ISSUES

Physical

- Have you considered your future life situation, personal values, and economic factors?
- How much is enough? E.g. what is the cost of success?
- Can you review and revise your financial plan: risk assessment, performance thresholds and automated alarms?
- Do you have a will, and Power of Attorney arrangements?
- Have you planned for your children if something happened to you?
- How much would you like to receive this year? Passive/worked
- How could you reduce your expenses? E.g. less entertainment/ gadgets/ education/ holidays/ health expenses/ pay off debts
- How could you increase your income? E.g. Work smarter/invest in shares or real estate

- Can you develop your financial future goals: E.g. annuities options/asset allocation/combine superannuation/further develop education/insurance/real estate's/retirement accounts/risk tolerance/roll over investments/savings plan/stock/tax strategies?
- Can you plan for a 'backup strategy' for your finances? E.g. identify alternative course of action, listen to others' recommendations, read over comprehensive written reports, seek out alternative financial advice
- Where can you save time or money E.g. what are all the opportunities, possibilities or hidden costs involved?

Mental

- Do you have in place who would care for all of the legal work related to the work you do? E.g. work contracts, intellectual property, copyrights and patents
- Do you read about financial information from a variety of sources? E.g. Reports/magazine/social media
- Are you conservative or a risk taker? E.g. the best way to predict your future is to create it?
- Are you prepared for financial success?

Emotional

- How are you going to react to getting future financial mail? E.g. Does getting bills in the mail or electronically scare you because you are running away from them?
- Do you have the courage to follow your financial dreams?
- Have you worked through the emotional blocks you have about financial success?

Spiritual

- How are you going to clear your money blocks: E.g. lack/ greed/ prosperity/ worthiness?
- Do you judge each day by the harvest you reap, instead of by the seeds you plant for the future?
- Do you feel you have a worthy purpose which keeps you on track?
- Can you invest in spiritual values/charities physically and emotionally?

Nutritional

- Will you spend money on good/organic/ethical food?
- Are you able to invest in your health? E.g. ethical, organic or free range food
- Can you build a garden or fund a community/school garden?
- Do you comply with all labelling laws for nutritional supplements you offer?
- Do you comply with laws around the nutritional advice you offer or essential oils you recommend?

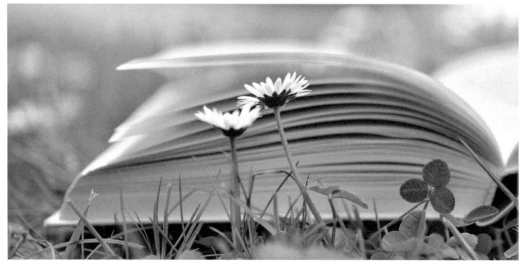

Physical

- What does your body want more of?
- What does your body want less of?
- Can you do more physical activities make you feel alive?
- How can you improve your physical movement to prevent diseases such as high blood pressure/heart disease/diabetes/obesity and improve mood?
- How can you exercise to increase endorphins, serotonin and dopamine, as well as release adrenaline? Life begins at the end of your comfort zone

Mental

- What health goals will bring you peace of mind? E.g. How we think directly influences our physical body

Emotional

- What health goals will give you your greatest level of emotional well-being? E.g. Exercising releases happy hormones

Spiritual

- How can you stay connected to your body? E.g. Know how your digestive/hormonal/skeletal/muscular/respiratory/immune system feels?
- Do you look after your spiritual body? E.g. run meridians, tai chi, yoga, chi gong
- Do you clear negative energy patterns that are either draining?
- Do you pay daily attention to the health of your aura/light bodies/chakras and other energy bodies?

Nutritional

- Can you eat the kind of foods that makes your body feel energised more regularly?
- Can you eat a balanced diet of protein/carbohydrates/fats and water consistently?
- Can you allow food to be your medicine and medicine be your food
- How can you support local farmers? E.g. buy direct, farmers markets, farmers co-ops

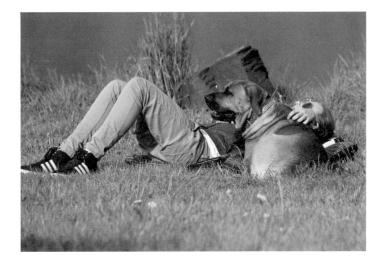

Life Balance

SPIRITUALITY

Physical

- How can you look after your body to have a better connection to your spirituality
- Can you eat more whole foods? Because the spirit is life, the mind is the builder, the physical is the result
- Can you do a physical exercise to suit your spiritual beliefs?

Mental

- Can you make peace with your past?
- Can you rule your mind? E.g. positive thoughts create a positive environment

Emotional

- Can you heal your emotions to allow for a freer future?
- Can you look at the cause of your emotions and not the symptoms? This will allow true healing of past wounds allowing for a calmer future

Spiritual

- Can you be receptive to a mentor? E.g. When the student is ready the teacher appears
- Can you realise more and more that everything is connected to everything? E.g. Every thought, action and reaction has a ripple effect
- Can you release the physical needs and ego? We are spiritual beings having a physical experience
- Can you connect more deeply into your spirituality?
- Can you say positive affirmations regularly?

Nutritional

- Can you bless all things living?
- Do you give thanks for the food you eat?
- Can you plant seeds of intention?
- Can you walk bare footed on the ground to reconnect to earth daily?

LIFE STYLE & HOUSING

Physical

- Can your home reflect your personality?
- Can your house be tidier inside and out? Do you need to de-clutter?
- Can you delegate what you don't have time for or what you don't like to do around the house?
- Can you include the family to all 'chip in' with domestic duties?

Mental

- Can you create a home that allows you to feel relaxed?
- Can you say 'I have enough material belongings"?
- Do you have a list of things you can do when you feel flat or lack energy?

Emotional

- Do you feel safe in your home to express your emotions?
- Are all emotions shared in the house? The good, the bad, and the ugly

Spiritual

- Can you create your own space/sanctuary in your house that you can be quiet/reflective in?

- Does your home have good Feng Shui and is it organised around your highest needs?

Nutritional

- Can you create a garden of any size at your house?
- How do you store your food so it stays fresh for longer?
- How important is purchasing organic food weekly to you?
- Can you grow a 'pretty' garden?

PAID WORK

Physical

- Can you organise your calendar by putting the big blocks in first, so the important is not overwhelmed by the urgent? Can you claim your calendar before someone else does? E.g. Time block in this order: birthday and holiday, holidays, industry events, vacations, board meetings, business review and staff meetings, special trips, time with friends, reviewing your life plan, other things that are important to you
- How can you get paid for a fair day's work?
- Are you aiming to climb the workplace ladder? What does it take to reach your goals?
- How can your physical requirements be met at work? E.g. safety/eco/movement
- Are you paying off your debts as quickly as possible?
- Are you planning for retirement with every pay packet?

Mental

- Can you prioritise your goals? E.g. Before things in our business life get busy
- Can you leave work at work in order to stay fresh with new ideas?
- Can you follow up on work projects to see the end results?
- Can you finish work ahead of time?
- What can you de-clutter? E.g. trash/add to a someday or maybe file/do it immediately/defer and reschedule/delegate
- Can you make your review of your week more efficient? E.g. follow-ups or thank you notes or a gift of appreciation
- Can you review your up-coming week on Sunday night? You may need to prepared or bring something to the event or finish a task before hand
- Can you review your pending list? It may be a list of items you have delegated out but still need to follow up on by an email or phoning
- Can you review your project list and consider the next action step required to keep the ball rolling in the future
- Can you review the someday/maybe list? E.g. this is the space where you park new ideas for projects of one day
- Does your combined work contribute positively to your mental well-being?
- Is your work mentally stimulating vs. boring or mentally exhausting?

Emotional

- How can you create a more positive environment at work? E.g. social club, raffles, BBQ's
- Can you create a playful environment? E.g. People who are creative have less sick days at work

Spiritual

- Can you give gratitude for the work you have and the blessings it provides you?
- Do you have an understanding of the spiritual meaning of your employment for the future?
- When you look around your workplace – does it bring you a sense of spiritual peace?

Life Balance

Nutritional

- Can you sit to eat?
- Can you create a pleasant space to relax and eat your food at work?
- Can you work and carry a water bottle with you at work?

NON – PAID WORK

Physical

- Can you make a positive impact on your community?
- Can you help the environment?
- What causes call you most deeply?
- How much money will you like to donate to charity? Which charity?

Mental

- Can you regularly send positive thoughts out into the community? Your love can change the outcome
- Can you refuse to support what doesn't resonate with your core beliefs? E.g. switch the TV off/don't give an opinion
- Can you stand for peace instead of justice?
- Does your non-paid work contribute positively to your mental well-being?
- Is your non-paid work mentally stimulating vs. boring or mentally exhausting?

Emotional

- Can you donate your time and heart to community project?
- Can you do regular random acts of kindness?
- Can you sponsor a child/animal/cause that is dear to your heart?

Spiritual

- Can you continually ask, "How could I do something to help change the world to be a better place"? E.g. prayer/gratitude/bless

Nutritional

- Can you plant a tree? How many and where?
- Can you connect with others at community gardens?
- Can you cook for others?

LIFE LONG LEARNING & DEVELOPMENT

Physical

- What would relax and inspire you?
- Can your bedroom be a tech free zone time without electronic devices?
- Can you take everything you need to create & stay focused for learning?
- Can you write your eulogy, what you would like to be remembered for? E.g. what you would pass on physically/traditions/knowledge
- What would bring more quality into your life? E.g. activities/relationships/habits

Mental

- How can you create the greatest impact in your learnings? How would you apply them?
- How could you stay open minded? E.g. what you know, what you know you don't know, what you don't know you don't know
- Can you connect with why your envisioned future is personally compelling?
- Can you de-clutter a busy mind? How?
- Can you stay clear on what is your retirement or legacy you are aiming to leave?
- Can you develop a passion for language and culture?
- What new programs of learning can you add to your life to keep yourself mentally engaged?

Emotional

- Can you listen to the whispers of your heart?
- Could you dream, imagine and create?
- Can you give thanks daily?
- What personal development programs can you do to increase your emotional wellbeing?

Spiritual

- Can you give yourself permission to learn something new every day?
- Can you give yourself days off that are good for the soul?
- Can meditation be a lifelong practise?
- How could you continually develop boundaries whilst expanding your compassion?
- Can you learn new spiritual practices to enhance your peace of mind?

Nutritional

- Can you learn about an area of nutrition that interests you?

MAKE IT HAPPEN!

Congratulations you have taken the time to decide what is really important for you in creating the lifestyle you really want. Now take the time to figure out your top priorities and schedule them into your diary. If they are in your schedule, there is a much greater chance that you will bring your dreams into reality. Organise your calendar, prioritise! Protect the basics (personal/family/health/spiritual time) eliminate the unnecessary and reschedule the rest.

REVIEW

Achieving your goals depends on giving them regular attention, connecting each goal from your head to your heart.

Take the time every 4/6/12 months to review the goals you set yourself

- What have you achieved? Congratulate yourself for your progress
- What goals have slipped by?
- Why?
- Are they still important?
- What can you do about it?
- Have your priorities changed? You can change your goals at any time.

It's your life. Have fun creating the life you have always dreamed of.

Life Balance

BUDGET PLANNER

This worksheet will assist you to identify your current cost of living.

Household Expenses

Rent/Water		Electricity and Gas		Rates/ Body Corporate Fees	
Telephone/Mobile		Cable/ TV/Internet		Furniture/ Appliances	
Cleaning/ Pool/Gardening					
Subtotal – Household				$	

Food

Groceries		Lunches		Restaurants & Takeaways	
Meat/ Fruit/ Vegetables				Pet food	
Subtotal – Food				$	

Personal Expenses

Clothes & Shoes		Hair & Beauty		Other	
Subtotal – Personal Expenses				$	

Medical Expenses

Doctor		Dentist		Specialist/ Therapies	
Chemist		Optometrist		Vet/Pet	
Subtotal – Medical Expenses				$	

Transport Expenses

Registration		Fuel		Public Transport	
Parking/Toll		Repairs/ Maintenance		Car Club Fees	
Subtotal – Transport Expenses				$	

Insurance

Home & Contents		Boat/Caravan		Life/TDP/Trauma	
Motor Vehicle		Health		Income Protection	
Rental Property		Other			
Subtotal – Insurance				$	

Other Expenses

Child Support Payments		Donations		Subscriptions, Magazines, Papers, Music, Movies	
Gifts – Christmas/Other		Hobbies & Sports/Gym		Alcohol & Cigarettes	
Holiday & Travel		Other Pet Costs		Lottery & Gaming	
Entertainment		Laundry/ Dry Cleaning		Children	
Special Projects		Other			
Subtotal – Other Expenses				$	

Savings

Superannuation Contribution		Regular savings		Regular Investments	
Subtotal – Savings				$	

Debt Repayment

Mortgage		Debt Repayment		Car Loan	
HECS/HELP Payments		Finance Companies		Credit Cards/ Store Cards	
Personal Loans		Lease/ Hire Purchase		Investment Loan	
Subtotal – Debt Repayment				$	

Investment Property

Loan Repayment		Agency Costs		Property Repairs	
Other Expenditure					
Subtotal – Other Expenses				$	

Education Expenses

School/university/ TAFE fees		Tuition/Lessons		Books & Uniforms	
Camps/Excursions				Child Care/Minding	

Subtotal – Education Expenses	$

INCOME

Section A Income	Yearly	Monthly / 12	Weekly /52
Income (After Tax)			
Your Net Income (After Tax)			
Partner/ Spouse Income (After Tax)			
Pension/ Benefit			
Family Payment			
Child Support Received			
Board Money Received			
Investments (After Tax)			
Other Income (After Tax)			
TOTAL INCOME (After Tax)			

LIVING EXPENSES

Section B Income	Yearly	Monthly / 12	Weekly /52
Household Expenses			
Food			
Personal Expenses			
Medical Expenses			
Transport Expenses			
Insurance			
Other Expenses			
Savings			
Investment Property			
Education Expenses			

TOTAL LIVING EXPENSES			

LOAN EXPENSES

Section C Income	Yearly	Monthly / 12	Weekly /52
Mortgage Expenses			
HECS/HELP Payments			
Personal Loans			
Debt Repayment			
Finance Companies			
Lease/ Hire Purchase			
Car Loan			
Credit Cards/ Store Cards			
Investment Loan			
TOTAL LOAN EXPENSES			

YOUR FINANCIAL SUMMARY

Total of Sections	Yearly	Monthly / 12	Weekly /52
TOTAL INCOME (After Tax) (From Section A)			
TOTAL LIVING EXPENSES (From Section B)			
TOTAL LOAN EXPENSES (From Section C)			
EQUALS EITHER SUPRPLUS (In Blue) or Deficit (In Red)			

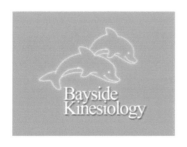

CONTACT
Bayside Kinesiology Brisbane,
Queensland AUSTRALIA

http://www.baysidekinesiology.com
ranee.zeller@baysidekinesiology.com

PH: 0419 737 396

REFERENCE

www.business.qld.gov.au/running-business/marketing-sales/marketing
promotion/advertising/unique-proposition
www.atms.com.au
www.articles.bplans.com
www.facebook.com
www.leadersinheels.com
www.mplans.com
www.tutorsglobe.com
www.entrepreneur.com
www.slideshare.net
www.documents.tips
www.studymoose.com
www.strategicmanagementinsight.com
www.davidmccrackenseo.com
www.dreamthisday.com
www.fakebuddhaquotes.com
www.industryweek.com
www.apple.com

SPECIAL THANK YOU

To my husband Bill, for putting up with me during my endless hours of research, my two kids, my parents and dear friends, for all their words of wisdom, editing and especially Belinda from 'Simply Designed for You' for her patience and graphic designing. To all my colleagues and professionals in the medical and natural therapy worlds who continuously give me other perspectives. Thank you to all my kinesiology teachers along the way, especially Philip Rafferty, founder of Kinergetics. Thank you to everyone for believing, supporting and encouraging me to see it through to publication. I thoroughly enjoy bringing facts to you in a simple, non-complicated way.

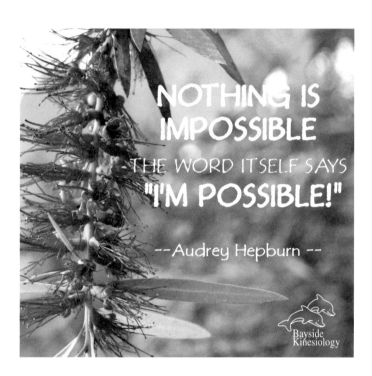

CONCLUSION

The aim of developing my 'HOW TO Kinesiology?' series was to bring my style of kinesiology into the homes of people and healers worldwide. This comprehensive guide covers everything you will need to know to begin balancing energy, in a quick and easy-to-understand format.

In conjunction with my series release, I have also developed a 5-day intensive course for 'HOW TO: Kinesiology?' As an Internationally registered course with the International Institute for Complementary Therapists, 'HOW TO: Kinesiology?' will give you the skills and training needed to better work with your own family — or clients in a clinical setting.

While it is not a requirement, I do recommend attending my course 'HOW TO: Kinesiology?' In a relaxed teaching environment, I will instruct you on how to clear your own stresses, fine tune your skills and become a stronger channel for correcting energy imbalances.

If I have started you on your journey of self-discovery or helped you along your life's path, my job is done.

Namaste

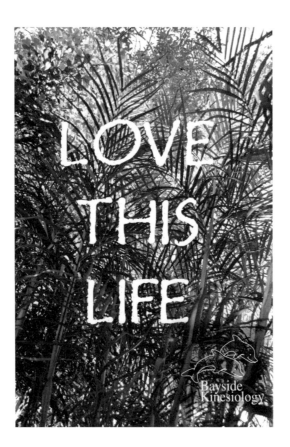

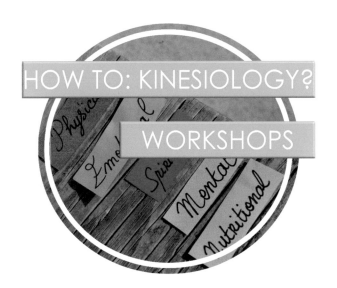

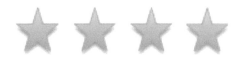

"Kinesiology for the office or the park!"
Amy B.

★ ★ ★ ★

"Comprehensive yet succinct"
Karen O'S.

HOW TO KINESIOLOGY? COURSES

- Abundance & Business Management
- Allergies
- Learning Enhancement
- Physical Pain & Fitness
- Spiritual Development
- Relationships & Love
- Nutrition & Weight Management
- Face Reading
- Meridians Made Easy

Don't forget these courses are also available via correspondence!

"One of the key 'go to' books in anyone's practice." Kaylene B.

"Easy to understand for beginners and the course provides videos to explain different techniques" Katie R.

Loads of Extras

- Peaceful eco-learning environment
- Increase your intuition/develop your questioning skills
- Live-in accommodation + airport pickups available

Trained & Qualified by The Founder, Ranee Zeller

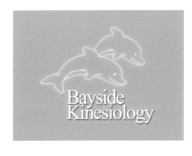

Other Courses

- Jaw R.E.S.E.T.
- Kinergetics

CONTACT

Bayside Kinesiology Brisbane, Queensland AUSTRALIA

Ph 0419 737 396

Web http//www.baysidekinesiology.com

Email ranee.zeller@baysidekinesiology.com

FOLLOW US!

Facebook	@BaysideKinesiology
YouTube	@BaysideKinesiology
Twitter	@BaysideKinesiol
Instagram	@BaysideKinesiology

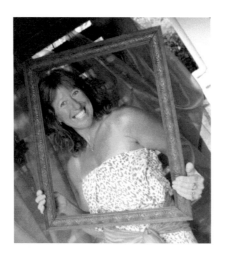

Calling all Kinesiologists dreaming of providing heart-felt kinesiology sessions that easily provide your clients with answers and direction...

The HOW TO: Kinesiology? series provides step-by-step kinesiology instructions.

Each of the 10 manuals is topic specific, covering the most popular concerns of clients.

For example money, relationships, weight management, allergies, learning problems, pain issues and spirituality.

To Purchase each manual is available as paperback, spiral or Epub.

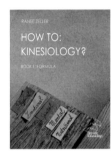

Book 1: Formula
Are you interested in learning how to apply kinesiology or are you already a Kinesiologist looking to improve your techniques?

My book 1 "Formula", from my book series "HOW TO Kinesiology", can give you all that.

This book is the foundation manual that puts the series together.
It includes:
- Written and video instruction on how to muscle test
- A kinesiology treatment protocol
- Verbal skills to prompt you on how to ask the right questions
- A list of correction solutions to make life easy for you
- Over 80 pages of scan lists for identifying the cause of issues, be it physical, mental, emotional, spiritual or nutritional

This manual is highly recommended if buying any of the other manuals in the series.

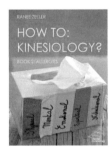

Book 2: Allergies
Do you suffer from allergies? Are you sick of taking pills? Would you like to find the cause and not just treat the symptoms?

Book 2 "Allergies" From the HOW TO: Kinesiology? Series gives you all that.

This manual provides:
- Over 100 pages of scan lists that focus on the cause of allergies, irritations or reactions
- It identifies environmental, natural, and man-made toxics that may have been ingested, inhaled, applied or injected
- It includes a BONUS client handout section for coeliac, milk, salicylate and nut dietary needs

This reference book works well with the first HOW TO Kinesiology? Book 1: Formula manual.

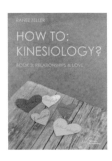

Book 3: Relationships and Love

Are you getting enough out of your relationship? Are you afraid that you are missing out on love? Are you looking for your secret love formula?

My kinesiology book "Relationships and Love" is a unique publication, which can help you with that.

It begins by looking at personal beliefs around love, goal setting and the five love languages.
It includes:
• A relationship questionnaire which highlights the physical, mental, emotional, spiritual and nutritional aspects of a number of love and relationship topics
• Identifies beliefs, sabotages, sexual concerns and more

The manual finishes with correction strategies, homework, intimacy ideas, and appendices on the Female and Male Reproductive Systems and the Anatomy of Orgasm.

Find your formula in 50 pages of a workbook!

This manual can be used alone or enhanced with the first book of the HOW TO: Kinesiology? Series.

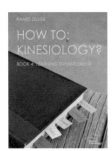

Book 4: Learning Enhancement

Are you still experiencing challenges with learning?
My kinesiology book "Learning Enhancement" can help you.
This manual was created for people of all ages and walks of life, to help with memory retention and the ability to process information.
The cause of that may come from genetic or social experiences and even gut intolerances

Once you have learned the foundations of kinesiology through my Book 1: Formula manual, book 4 guides you or your client back to learning enhancement.

It is a complete learning package and includes scan lists from physical, mental, emotional, spiritual and nutritional details.

This book can be used alone if the user is experienced with muscle testing. If not, the first book of the HOW TO: Kinesiology? series is recommended.

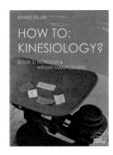

Book 5: Nutrition and Weight Management

Are you experiencing problems with your weight? Too much or too little?

Or are you a Kinesiologist who dreams of specializing in nutrition and weight management?

My kinesiology book "Nutrition and Weight Management" can help you with that.

This extremely thought provoking manual provides a well-rounded approach to health and vitality with questions such as:

- Is the nutrition able to be digested, assimilated, metabolized or eliminated?
- Is the nutritional problem environmental, genetic, man-made, toxic overload or emotional?

It's a complete package and includes physical, mental, emotional, spiritual and nutritional scan lists as well as overviews to vitamins, minerals, heavy metals, diet types and much, much more.

Included is 12 BONUS client handouts including Coeliac, Dairy, Paleo, Ayurvedic, Blood type, Tasting and more.

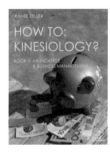

Book 6: Abundance and Business Management

Do you want freedom to move forward with your personal life and business goals? Are you ready to step into prosperity?

My kinesiology manual "Abundance and Business Management" can help you with that.

We realise that somewhere in the future you want to see yourself living a fulfilling life while working in a thriving business. We know you've got an internal image of yourself, of the impact you want to make in the world, and the people you want to serve.

I know when you get to the end of your life and look back you will wish that you had had the biggest impact.

This book includes tools for attracting abundance which is authentic to you. While aimed at therapists, it is valuable for all people wanting to improve their business and life skills.

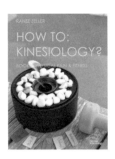

Book 7: Physical Pain and Fitness

Are you in physical pain? Or do you want to improve your fitness? My kinesiology manual "Physical Pain and Fitness" can help you with that.

It has everything in one book for the athletic to the 'less' active as well as the chronic fatigue client.

As a therapist with the relevant scan lists in the categories of physical, mental, emotional, spiritual, and nutritional you can start to rebuild and reprogram a healthy body.

Included in this manual are comprehensive lists on muscles and bones, posture, breathing techniques, injury prevention, risk management, recovery strategies, gym terms as well as developing a training program.

This book can be used alone if the user is experienced with muscle testing. If not, the first book of the HOW TO: Kinesiology? series is recommended.

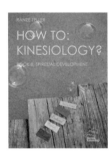

Book 8: Spiritual Development

Are you looking for spirituality? Do you want to bring this into your kinesiology clinic with confidence?

This book is not a book on how to find enlightenment but rather a book that offers a faster road to clearing fears which may be holding you back. It also gives simple meanings for spiritual words, experiences and entities.

With over 160 pages the "Spiritual Development" book offers an extended explanation of the spiritual scan lists provided in the HOW TO: Kinesiology? Book 1: Formula.

While aimed at therapists, it is valuable for all people wanting to travel and explore the world of spirituality.

This book can be used alone if the user is experienced with muscle testing. If not, the first book of the HOW TO: Kinesiology? series is recommended for a complete package.

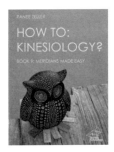

Book 9: Meridians Made Easy

Are you interested in meridian and energy lines?

My "Meridians Made Easy" reference book provides easy-to-find information on the meridians. It is a must-have for every Kinesiologist as it provides one concise page for each meridian including common disorders, pictures of the meridians, muscles affected, relevant questions for related disorders, neurovascular and neurolymphatic reflex points, yin/yang, number of acupuncture points, time of day function, element, season, astrological sign, body system, colour, sound, fluid and emotional states.

This book can be used alone if the user is experienced with muscle testing. If not, the first book of the HOW TO: Kinesiology? series is recommended for a complete package.

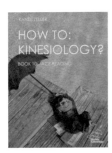

Book 10: Face Reading

Do you want to learn how to read people's faces?

My kinesiology manual "Face Reading" shows you how.

Face reading has multiple facets; once you can read a person's facial features you can understand the automatic behaviours and silent messages of the soul.

This book covers:
- The most common traits and includes diagrams and explanations
- Employment opportunities and challenges relating to each feature
- Use this technique of face reading to sum up a client before designing a treatment program tailor made for them

Manuals 2 – 10 are great stand-alone reference books for the healer. The first book of the HOW TO: Kinesiology? series is recommended for a complete package.

Made in United States
Troutdale, OR
10/03/2024

23391496R00079